Fix Your Body Mechanics

Also by Ya-Ling J. Liou D.C.

Put Out the Fire: "It Never Used to Hurt When I...?!"
(The Everyday Pain Guide, Volume 1)

Fix the Fire Damage: Your go-to guide when pain first strikes
(The Everyday Pain Guide, Volume 2)

Fix Your Body Mechanics: Companion Manual & Journal
(The Everyday Pain Guide Workbooks #1)

Fix Your Body Chemistry: Companion Manual & Journal
(The Everyday Pain Guide Workbooks #2)

Fix Your Stress Biology: Companion Manual & Journal
(The Everyday Pain Guide Workbooks #3)

The Everyday Pain Guide
WORKBOOKS

VOL.2
FIX THE
FIRE DAMAGE!

Fix Your Body Mechanics

COMPANION MANUAL & JOURNAL

YA-LING J. LIOU, D.C.

Artwork by SANDY JOHNSON

RETURN TO HEALTH PRESS
SEATTLE, WA

FIX YOUR BODY MECHANICS COMPANION MANUAL & JOURNAL
(THE EVERYDAY PAIN GUIDE WORKBOOKS #1)
© 2025 Ya-Ling J. Liou, D.C.
All rights reserved.

Published by Return to Health Press, Seattle, WA
Ya-Ling J. Liou, D.C., is a chiropractic physician in Seattle, WA
www.returntohealthpress.com

Notice
The information, techniques and suggestions contained in this book are not intended as a substitute for individual medical care. All matters regarding your health require medical supervision. Consult your health care professional before performing any exercise or taking any dietary supplement referenced in this book. Neither the author, nor the publisher, contributors or editors shall be liable or responsible for any loss, damage or risk arising, directly or indirectly, from the use and application of any of the contents of this book.

Cover Design by VMC Art & Design, LLC
Interior Design by VMC Art & Design, LLC
Image & Diagram Credits: 1983 Wong-Baker FACES Foundation. www.wongbakerfaces.org

First Edition, 2025
Printed in the United States of America

ISBN: 978-0-9913094-4-3

CONTENTS

Author's Note

For best results, make sure to seek care as soon as possible and/or in conjunction with these strategies. Always check with a healthcare provider first.

SURPRISE PAIN?

Neck/Shoulder

Mid Back/Torso/Ribs

Neck

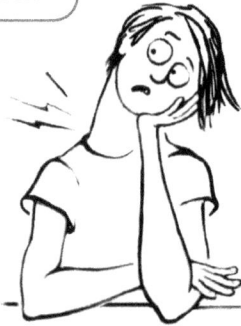 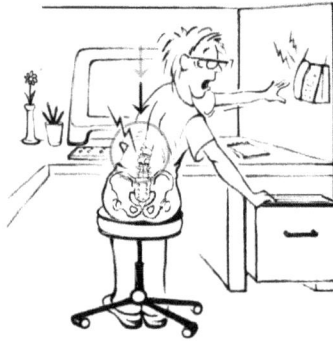 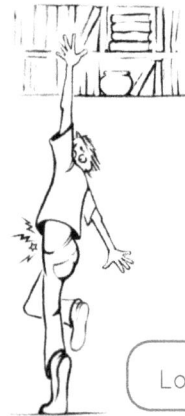

Low Back

Shoulder/Upper Back

Hip/Buttock/Thigh

Low Back/Hip

➜ BODY MECHANICS ACTION PLANS

☑ BODY CHEMISTRY ACTION PLAN

☑ STRESS BIOLOGY ACTION PLAN

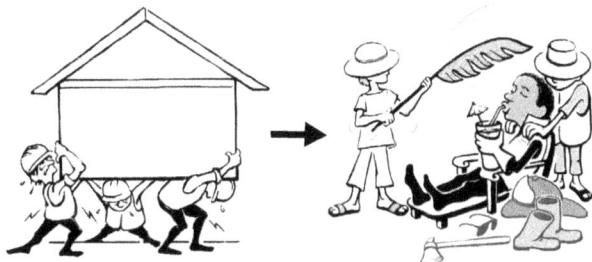

1. RELEASE

- **Mechanical Strain**
  - *Body Chemistry Garbage*
  - *Emotional Stress Triggers*

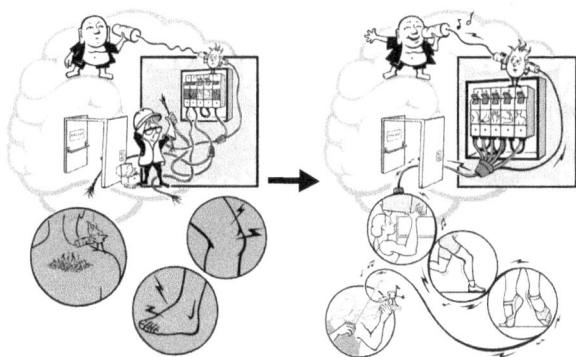

2. RETRAIN

- **Body-Brain Connection**
  - *Garbage Journeys*
  - *Nervous System*

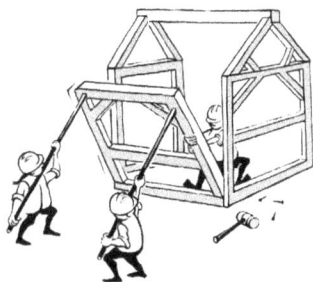

3. REINFORCE

- **Mechanical Structure**
  - *Garbage Elimination*
  - *Low-Stress Biology*

"To me, if life boils down to one thing, it's movement. To live is to keep moving."

—Jerry Seinfeld

My
Release
Action
Steps

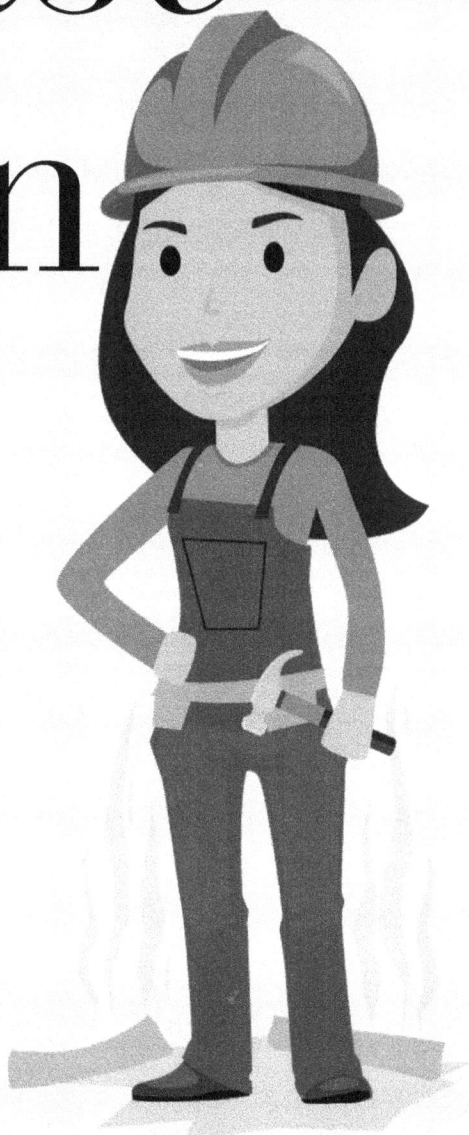

THE CHECK IN

How are you feeling?

TODAY'S DATE: _____

PAIN LOCATION:
(circle one)

Neck   Neck/Shoulder   Shoulder/Upper Back   Mid Back/Torso/Ribs

Low Back   Low Back/Hip   Hip/Buttock/Thigh

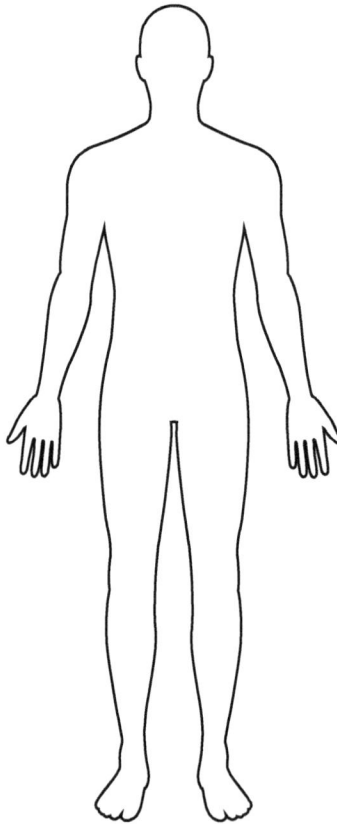

Use this figure to color or shade-in the area of your pain however you like.

HOW MUCH PAIN TODAY?

Circle the face below that best expresses your discomfort:

Wong-Baker FACES® Pain Rating Scale

0	2	4	6	8	10
No Pain	A Little Pain	A Little More Pain	Even More Pain	A Whole Lot Of Pain	Worst Pain

Notes:

_____

_____

_____

_____

_____

_____

_____

_____

_____

_____

My pain feels:
(circle all that apply)

Sharp   Stabbing   Achy   Tingly   Throbbing

Grabbing   Tightness   Pinching

Other/More Details: _____

_____

_____

_____

When do I notice it the *most*?
(circle all that apply)

Sitting   Standing still   Walking   Getting up from sitting

Lying on my back   Lying on my belly   Lying on my RIGHT side

Lying on my LEFT side   Driving the car   Mornings

Before bed   Middle of the night

Other/More Details: _____

_____

_____

_____

When do I notice it *less*?
(circle all that apply)

Sitting   Standing still   Walking   Getting up from sitting

Lying on my back   Lying on my belly   Lying on my RIGHT side

Lying on my LEFT side   Driving the car   Mornings

Before bed   Middle of the night

Other/More Details: _____

_____

_____

_____

_____

Medication used:
(circle all that apply)

Ibuprofen (Motrin/Advil)   Naproxen (Aleve)   Acetaminophen (Tylenol)

Other/Prescription: _____

_____

How much? _____

_____

☐ Some Relief?   ☐ Total Relief?   ☐ No Relief?

RELEASE!

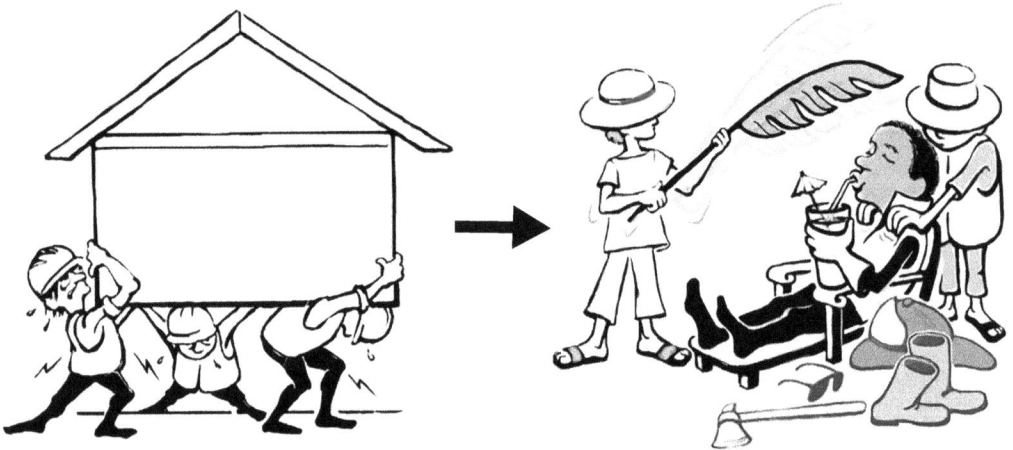

Before relief is possible, we must allow the protective (often pain causing) mechanisms to *release* their grip and calm down. To put out that fire of active inflammation, the best thing to do is to stop fueling the inflammation fire.

Q: *What* are you releasing?

A: Your nervous system's grip on the "soft tissues"—muscles and tendons

Q: *How* are you releasing your soft tissues?

A: Through neutralizing positioning and rest

NEXT STEPS:

1. Visit the Body Mechanics Action Plans in *The Everyday Pain Guide – Fix the Fire Damage* & find the action plan for your pain location.

2. Try all **Release** activities associated with your pain location.

3. Pick up to three **Release** activities for daily use as needed and record your progress each day using the following pages…

This first phase in any of the three Action Plans—Body Mechanics, Body Chemistry, and Stress Biology—is just as important for familiar recurring pain as it is when dealing with fresh and new pain.

The Release phase is where you will see exactly how to stop the fire of inflammation in its tracks. Following these steps in this section provides you with your body mechanics "stop, drop, and roll" moment which will allow the painful area(s)"on fire" to return to neutral and get a tiny, much needed break from the pain.

Notes:

_____

_____

_____

_____

_____

_____

_____

_____

_____

_____

_____

_____

_____

_____

_____

Release
Activities

Week One

RELEASE – DAY 1

TODAY'S DATE: _____

Pick up to three of the following RELEASE activities:

(Go to the Exercise Index in the Resources section at the back of the book, Fix the Fire Damage, to help you find these activities.)

- ☐ Lie down and support your neck

- ☐ Lie down and support your low back

- ☐ Lie down and support your low back + hip

- ☐ Sleep position strategy +/or posture reset

- ☐ Sleep position strategy face up

- ☐ Sleep position strategy side lying

- ☐ Sleep position strategy belly face down

- ☐ Partial Bruegger's Relief positioning

- ☐ Pendulum passive release

- ☐ Seated to standing transition

- ☐ Hip rotator release against the wall

- ☐ Modified sphinx pose

- ☐ Hamstring stretch

RELEASE ACTIVITIES

RELEASE Activity #1: _____

Better? _____   Worse? _____   Same? _____

Other: _____

Notes: _____

_____

RELEASE Activity #2: _____

Better? _____   Worse? _____   Same? _____

Other: _____

Notes: _____

_____

RELEASE Activity #3: _____

Better? _____   Worse? _____   Same? _____

Other: _____

Notes: _____

_____

PAIN LOCATION:

Use this figure to color or shade-in the area of your pain however you like.

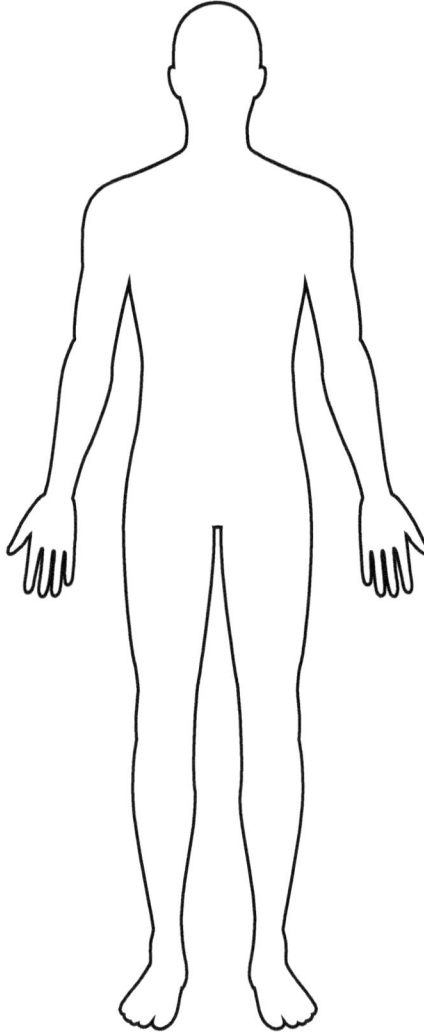

Quick Guide: Pain Locations

As seen in *The Everyday Pain Guide—Fix the Fire Damage*

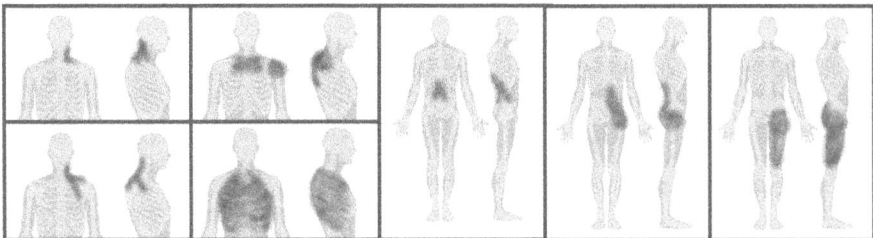

HOW MUCH PAIN TODAY?

Circle the face that best expresses your discomfort:

Wong-Baker FACES® Pain Rating Scale

0	**2**	**4**	**6**	**8**	**10**
No Pain	A Little Pain	A Little More Pain	Even More Pain	A Whole Lot Of Pain	Worst Pain

Notes:

_____

_____

_____

_____

_____

_____

_____

_____

Remember to check out the Release phases of body chemistry and stress biology action plans.

DAY 1 AFFIRMATION

Write it down. Say it out loud. Repeat often.

"I trust my body."

_____

_____

_____

_____

_____

_____

_____

_____

_____

_____

DAY 1 MINDSET MOJO

Food for thought. Try it.

Think of and speak of your pain in the past tense.

What does this bring up for you? Write about it. Free associate.

_____

_____

_____

_____

_____

_____

_____

_____

_____

_____

RELEASE - DAY 2

TODAY'S DATE: _____

Pick up to three of the following RELEASE activities:

(Go to the Exercise Index in the Resources section at the back of the book, Fix the Fire Damage, to help you find these activities.)

- [ ] Lie down and support your neck

- [ ] Lie down and support your low back

- [ ] Lie down and support your low back + hip

- [ ] Sleep position strategy +/or posture reset

- [ ] Sleep position strategy face up

- [ ] Sleep position strategy side lying

- [ ] Sleep position strategy belly face down

- [ ] Partial Bruegger's Relief positioning

- [ ] Pendulum passive release

- [ ] Seated to standing transition

- [ ] Hip rotator release against the wall

- [ ] Modified sphinx pose

- [ ] Hamstring stretch

RELEASE ACTIVITIES

RELEASE Activity #1: _____

Better? _____   Worse? _____   Same? _____

Other: _____

Notes: _____

_____

RELEASE Activity #2: _____

Better? _____   Worse? _____   Same? _____

Other: _____

Notes: _____

_____

RELEASE Activity #3: _____

Better? _____   Worse? _____   Same? _____

Other: _____

Notes: _____

_____

PAIN LOCATION:

Use this figure to color or shade-in the area of your pain however you like.

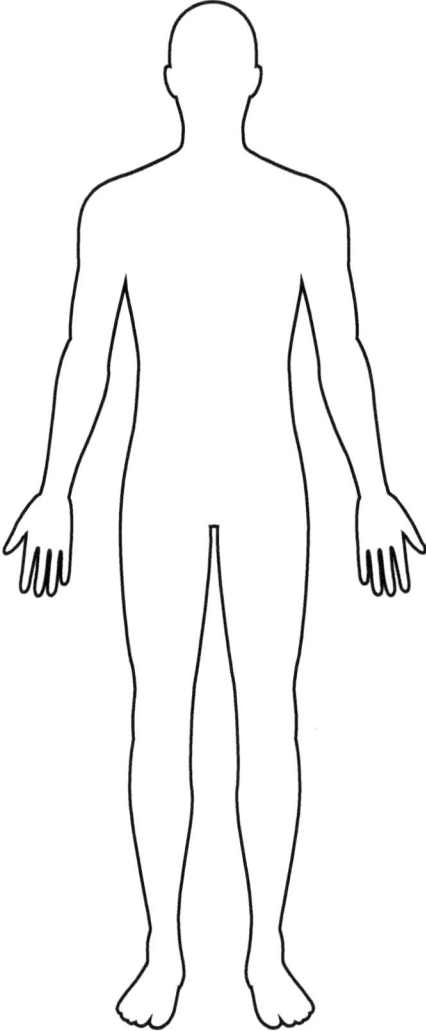

Quick Guide: Pain Locations

As seen in *The Everyday Pain Guide—Fix the Fire Damage*

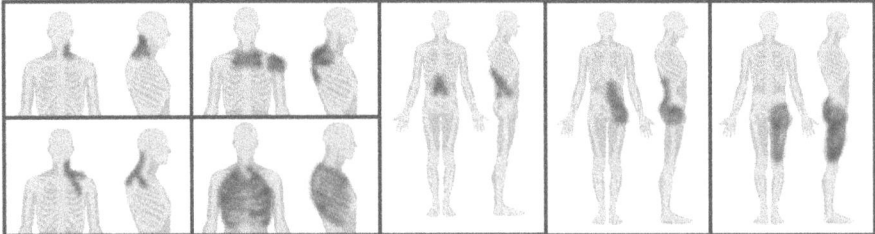

HOW MUCH PAIN TODAY?

Circle the face that best expresses your discomfort:

Wong-Baker FACES® Pain Rating Scale

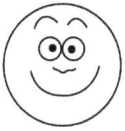 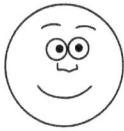 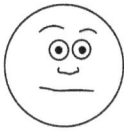 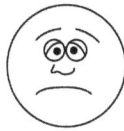 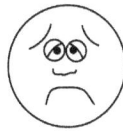 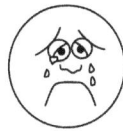

0	2	4	6	8	10
No Pain	A Little Pain	A Little More Pain	Even More Pain	A Whole Lot Of Pain	Worst Pain

Notes:

_____

_____

_____

_____

_____

_____

_____

Remember to check out the Release phases of body chemistry and stress biology action plans.

DAY 2 AFFIRMATION

Write it down. Say it out loud. Repeat often.

"My body is doing exactly what it's supposed to."

DAY 2 MINDSET MOJO

Food for thought. Try it.

Be kind to yourself!

What does this bring up for you? Write about it. Free associate.

_____

_____

_____

_____

_____

_____

_____

_____

_____

_____

RELEASE - DAY 3

TODAY'S DATE: _____

Pick up to three of the following RELEASE activities:

(Go to the Exercise Index in the Resources section at the back of the book, Fix the Fire Damage, to help you find these activities.)

- ☐ Lie down and support your neck

- ☐ Lie down and support your low back

- ☐ Lie down and support your low back + hip

- ☐ Sleep position strategy +/or posture reset

- ☐ Sleep position strategy face up

- ☐ Sleep position strategy side lying

- ☐ Sleep position strategy belly face down

- ☐ Partial Bruegger's Relief positioning

- ☐ Pendulum passive release

- ☐ Seated to standing transition

- ☐ Hip rotator release against the wall

- ☐ Modified sphinx pose

- ☐ Hamstring stretch

RELEASE ACTIVITIES

RELEASE Activity #1: _____

Better? _____   Worse? _____   Same? _____

Other: _____

Notes: _____

_____

RELEASE Activity #2: _____

Better? _____   Worse? _____   Same? _____

Other: _____

Notes: _____

_____

RELEASE Activity #3: _____

Better? _____   Worse? _____   Same? _____

Other: _____

Notes: _____

_____

PAIN LOCATION:

Use this figure to color or shade-in the area of your pain however you like.

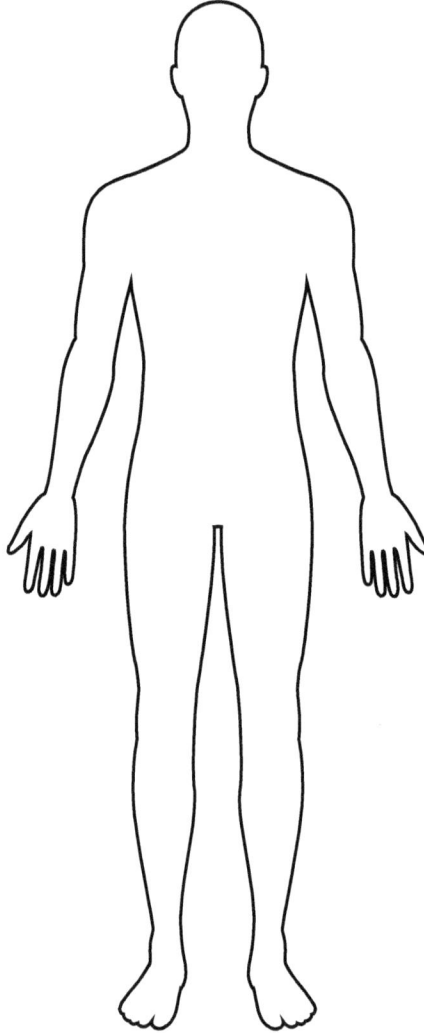

Quick Guide: Pain Locations

As seen in *The Everyday Pain Guide—Fix the Fire Damage*

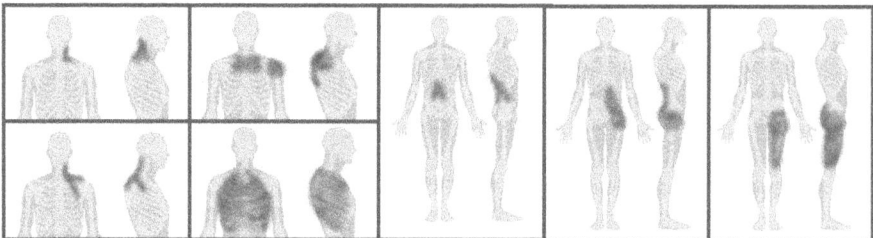

HOW MUCH PAIN TODAY?

Circle the face that best expresses your discomfort:

Wong-Baker FACES® Pain Rating Scale

0	2	4	6	8	10
No Pain	A Little Pain	A Little More Pain	Even More Pain	A Whole Lot Of Pain	Worst Pain

Notes:

_____

_____

_____

_____

_____

_____

_____

Remember to check out the Release phases of body chemistry and stress biology action plans.

DAY 3 AFFIRMATION

Write it down. Say it out loud. Repeat often.

"I have a strong and resilient body."

_____

_____

_____

_____

_____

_____

_____

_____

_____

DAY 3 MINDSET MOJO

Food for thought. Try it.

What happens when you listen to your pain?

What does this bring up for you? Write about it. Free associate.

_____

_____

_____

_____

_____

_____

_____

_____

_____

_____

RELEASE – DAY 4

TODAY'S DATE: _____

Pick up to three of the following RELEASE activities:

(Go to the Exercise Index in the Resources section at the back of the book, Fix the Fire Damage, to help you find these activities.)

- ☐ Lie down and support your neck

- ☐ Lie down and support your low back

- ☐ Lie down and support your low back + hip

- ☐ Sleep position strategy +/or posture reset

- ☐ Sleep position strategy face up

- ☐ Sleep position strategy side lying

- ☐ Sleep position strategy belly face down

- ☐ Partial Bruegger's Relief positioning

- ☐ Pendulum passive release

- ☐ Seated to standing transition

- ☐ Hip rotator release against the wall

- ☐ Modified sphinx pose

- ☐ Hamstring stretch

RELEASE ACTIVITIES

RELEASE Activity #1: _____

Better? _____   Worse? _____   Same? _____

Other: _____

Notes: _____

_____

RELEASE Activity #2: _____

Better? _____   Worse? _____   Same? _____

Other: _____

Notes: _____

_____

RELEASE Activity #3: _____

Better? _____   Worse? _____   Same? _____

Other: _____

Notes: _____

_____

PAIN LOCATION:

Use this figure to color or shade-in the area of your pain however you like.

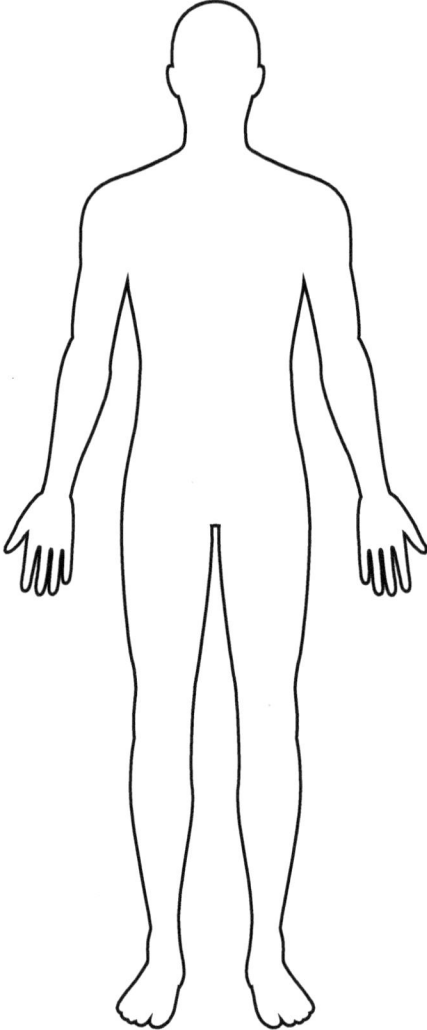

Quick Guide: Pain Locations

As seen in *The Everyday Pain Guide—Fix the Fire Damage*

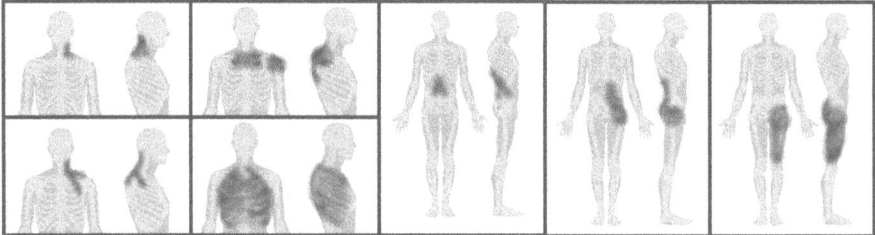

HOW MUCH PAIN TODAY?

Circle the face that best expresses your discomfort:

Wong-Baker FACES® Pain Rating Scale

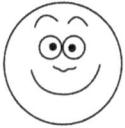 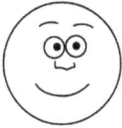 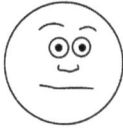 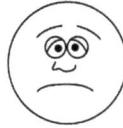 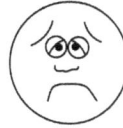 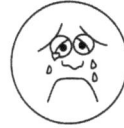

0	**2**	**4**	**6**	**8**	**10**
No Pain	A Little Pain	A Little More Pain	Even More Pain	A Whole Lot Of Pain	Worst Pain

Notes:

_____

_____

_____

_____

_____

_____

_____

Remember to check out the Release phases of body chemistry and stress biology action plans.

DAY 4 AFFIRMATION

Write it down. Say it out loud. Repeat often.

"My body knows just what to do."

DAY 4 MINDSET MOJO

Food for thought. Try it.

You did nothing wrong.

What does this bring up for you? Write about it. Free associate.

RELEASE – DAY 5

TODAY'S DATE: _____

Pick up to three of the following RELEASE activities:

(Go to the Exercise Index in the Resources section at the back of the book, Fix the Fire Damage, to help you find these activities.)

- ☐ Lie down and support your neck

- ☐ Lie down and support your low back

- ☐ Lie down and support your low back + hip

- ☐ Sleep position strategy +/or posture reset

- ☐ Sleep position strategy face up

- ☐ Sleep position strategy side lying

- ☐ Sleep position strategy belly face down

- ☐ Partial Bruegger's Relief positioning

- ☐ Pendulum passive release

- ☐ Seated to standing transition

- ☐ Hip rotator release against the wall

- ☐ Modified sphinx pose

- ☐ Hamstring stretch

RELEASE ACTIVITIES

RELEASE Activity #1: _____

Better? _____   Worse? _____   Same? _____

Other: _____

Notes: _____

_____

RELEASE Activity #2: _____

Better? _____   Worse? _____   Same? _____

Other: _____

Notes: _____

_____

RELEASE Activity #3: _____

Better? _____   Worse? _____   Same? _____

Other: _____

Notes: _____

_____

PAIN LOCATION:

Use this figure to color or shade-in the area of your pain however you like.

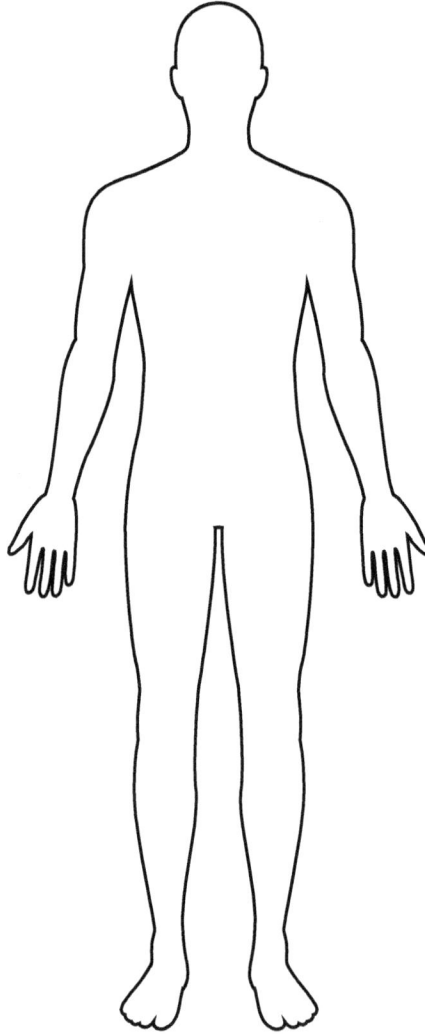

Quick Guide: Pain Locations

As seen in *The Everyday Pain Guide—Fix the Fire Damage*

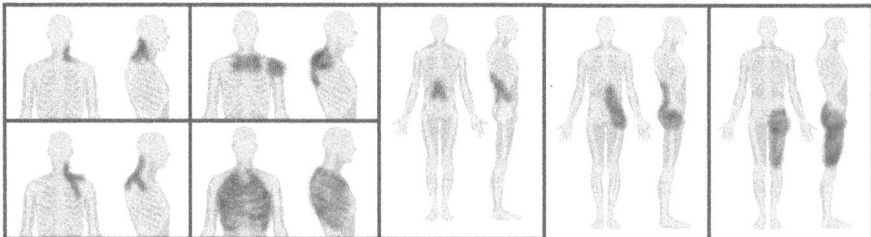

HOW MUCH PAIN TODAY?

Circle the face that best expresses your discomfort:

Wong-Baker FACES® Pain Rating Scale

0	2	4	6	8	10
No Pain	A Little Pain	A Little More Pain	Even More Pain	A Whole Lot Of Pain	Worst Pain

Notes:

_____

_____

_____

_____

_____

_____

_____

Remember to check out the Release phases of body chemistry and stress biology action plans.

DAY 5 AFFIRMATION

Write it down. Say it out loud. Repeat often.

"My pain is a sensible message and I'm listening."

_____

_____

_____

_____

_____

_____

_____

_____

_____

DAY 5 MINDSET MOJO

Food for thought. Try it.

You are doing your best
and that is enough.

What does this bring up for you? Write about it. Free associate.

_____

_____

_____

_____

_____

_____

_____

_____

_____

_____

RELEASE – DAY 6

TODAY'S DATE: _____

Pick up to three of the following RELEASE activities:

(Go to the Exercise Index in the Resources section at the back of the book, Fix the Fire Damage, to help you find these activities.)

☐ Lie down and support your neck

☐ Lie down and support your low back

☐ Lie down and support your low back + hip

☐ Sleep position strategy +/or posture reset

☐ Sleep position strategy face up

☐ Sleep position strategy side lying

☐ Sleep position strategy belly face down

☐ Partial Bruegger's Relief positioning

☐ Pendulum passive release

☐ Seated to standing transition

☐ Hip rotator release against the wall

☐ Modified sphinx pose

☐ Hamstring stretch

RELEASE ACTIVITIES

RELEASE Activity #1: _____

Better? _____   Worse? _____   Same? _____

Other: _____

Notes: _____

_____

RELEASE Activity #2: _____

Better? _____   Worse? _____   Same? _____

Other: _____

Notes: _____

_____

RELEASE Activity #3: _____

Better? _____   Worse? _____   Same? _____

Other: _____

Notes: _____

_____

PAIN LOCATION:

Use this figure to color or shade-in the area of your pain however you like.

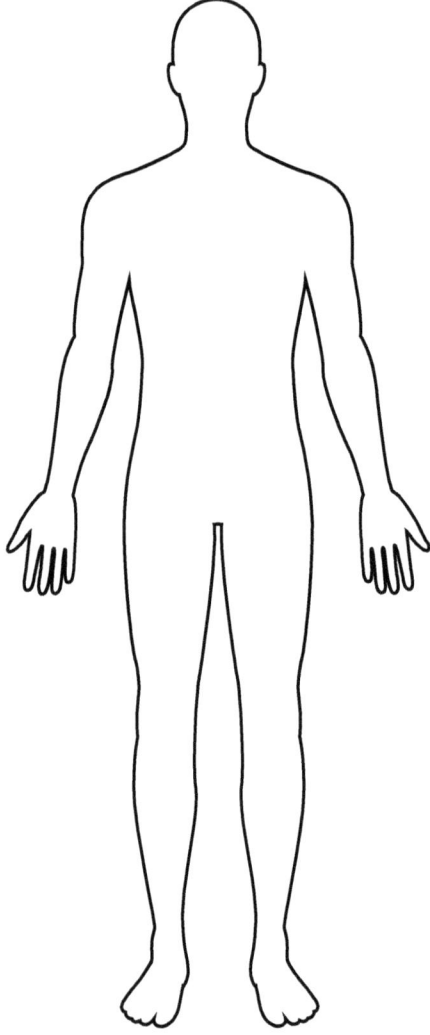

Quick Guide: Pain Locations

As seen in *The Everyday Pain Guide—Fix the Fire Damage*

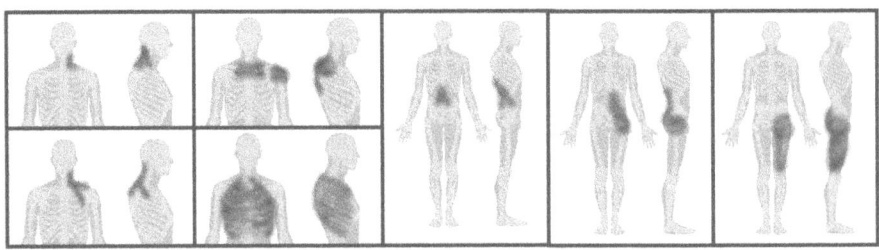

HOW MUCH PAIN TODAY?

Circle the face that best expresses your discomfort:

Wong-Baker FACES® Pain Rating Scale

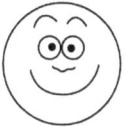 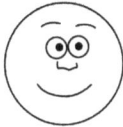 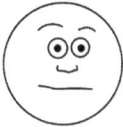 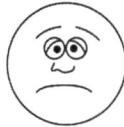 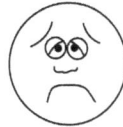 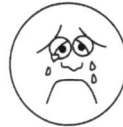

0	2	4	6	8	10
No Pain	A Little Pain	A Little More Pain	Even More Pain	A Whole Lot Of Pain	Worst Pain

Notes:

_____

_____

_____

_____

_____

_____

_____

Remember to check out the Release phases of body chemistry and stress biology action plans.

DAY 6 AFFIRMATION

Write it down. Say it out loud. Repeat often.

"My body is telling me something important about how to move forward into better health."

_____

_____

_____

_____

_____

_____

_____

_____

_____

_____

DAY 6 MINDSET MOJO

Food for thought. Try it.

Breathe.

What does this bring up for you? Write about it. Free associate.

_____

_____

_____

_____

_____

_____

_____

_____

_____

_____

RELEASE - DAY 7

TODAY'S DATE: _____

Pick up to three of the following RELEASE activities:

(Go to the Exercise Index in the Resources section at the back of the book, Fix the Fire Damage, to help you find these activities.)

☐ Lie down and support your neck

☐ Lie down and support your low back

☐ Lie down and support your low back + hip

☐ Sleep position strategy +/or posture reset

☐ Sleep position strategy face up

☐ Sleep position strategy side lying

☐ Sleep position strategy belly face down

☐ Partial Bruegger's Relief positioning

☐ Pendulum passive release

☐ Seated to standing transition

☐ Hip rotator release against the wall

☐ Modified sphinx pose

☐ Hamstring stretch

RELEASE ACTIVITIES

RELEASE Activity #1: _____

Better? _____   Worse? _____   Same? _____

Other: _____

Notes: _____

_____

RELEASE Activity #2: _____

Better? _____   Worse? _____   Same? _____

Other: _____

Notes: _____

_____

RELEASE Activity #3: _____

Better? _____   Worse? _____   Same? _____

Other: _____

Notes: _____

_____

PAIN LOCATION:

Use this figure to color or shade-in the area of your pain however you like.

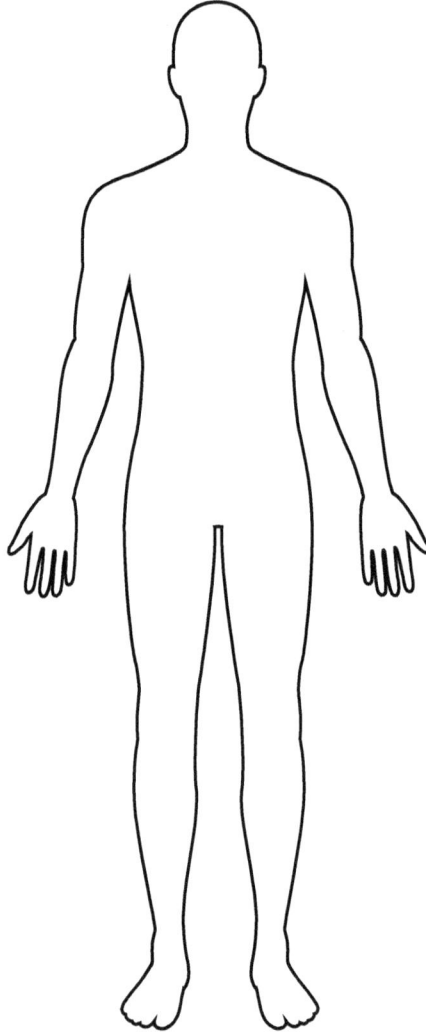

Quick Guide: Pain Locations

As seen in *The Everyday Pain Guide—Fix the Fire Damage*

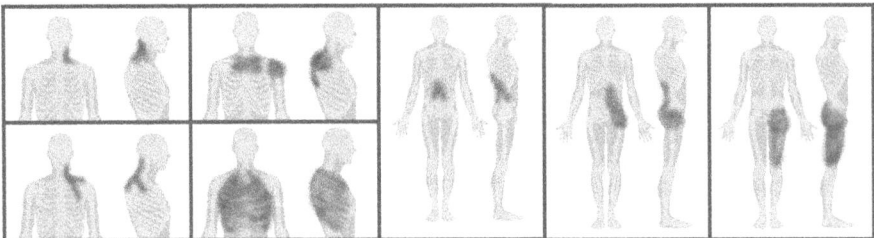

HOW MUCH PAIN TODAY?

Circle the face that best expresses your discomfort:

Wong-Baker FACES® Pain Rating Scale

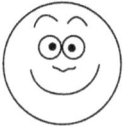 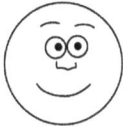 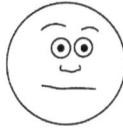 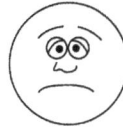 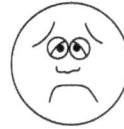 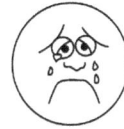

0	2	4	6	8	10
No Pain	A Little Pain	A Little More Pain	Even More Pain	A Whole Lot Of Pain	Worst Pain

Notes:

_____

_____

_____

_____

_____

_____

_____

Remember to check out the Release phases of body chemistry and stress biology action plans.

DAY 7 AFFIRMATION

Write it down. Say it out loud. Repeat often.

"My body is watching out for me and all is well."

DAY 7 MINDSET MOJO

Food for thought. Try it.

You are not alone.

What does this bring up for you? Write about it. Free associate.

_____

_____

_____

_____

_____

_____

_____

_____

_____

_____

Notes:

_____

_____

_____

_____

_____

_____

_____

_____

_____

_____

_____

_____

_____

_____

_____

Release Activities

Week Two

RELEASE – DAY 1

TODAY'S DATE: _____

Pick up to three of the following RELEASE activities:

(Go to the Exercise Index in the Resources section at the back of the book, Fix the Fire Damage, to help you find these activities.)

- ☐ Lie down and support your neck

- ☐ Lie down and support your low back

- ☐ Lie down and support your low back + hip

- ☐ Sleep position strategy +/or posture reset

- ☐ Sleep position strategy face up

- ☐ Sleep position strategy side lying

- ☐ Sleep position strategy belly face down

- ☐ Partial Bruegger's Relief positioning

- ☐ Pendulum passive release

- ☐ Seated to standing transition

- ☐ Hip rotator release against the wall

- ☐ Modified sphinx pose

- ☐ Hamstring stretch

RELEASE ACTIVITIES

RELEASE Activity #1: _____

Better? _____   Worse? _____   Same? _____

Other: _____

Notes: _____

_____

RELEASE Activity #2: _____

Better? _____   Worse? _____   Same? _____

Other: _____

Notes: _____

_____

RELEASE Activity #3: _____

Better? _____   Worse? _____   Same? _____

Other: _____

Notes: _____

_____

PAIN LOCATION:

Use this figure to color or shade-in the area of your pain however you like.

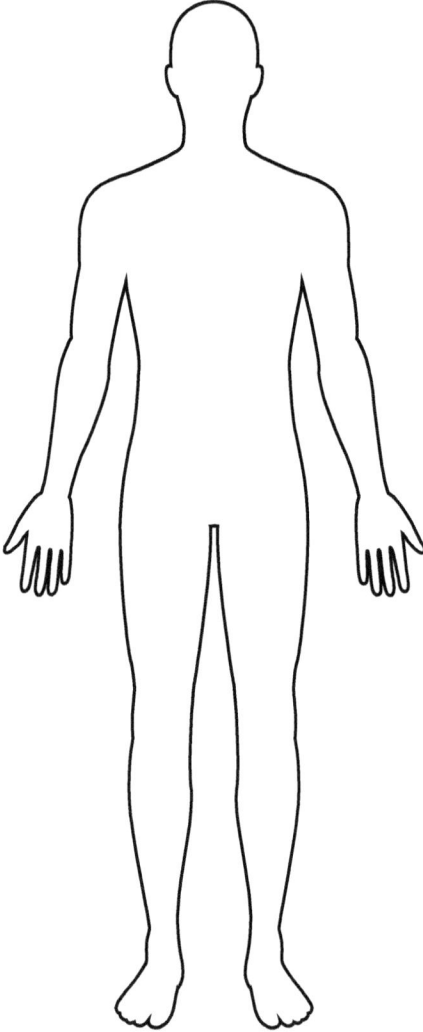

Quick Guide: Pain Locations

As seen in *The Everyday Pain Guide—Fix the Fire Damage*

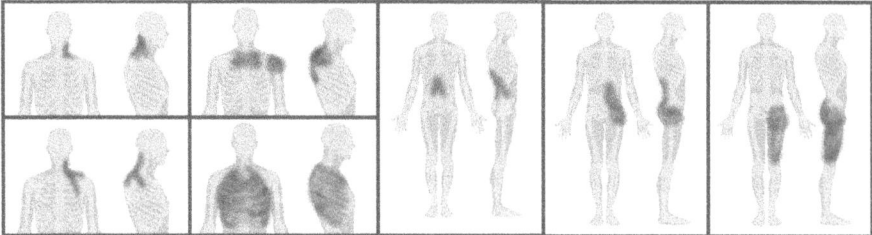

HOW MUCH PAIN TODAY?

Circle the face that best expresses your discomfort:

Wong-Baker FACES® Pain Rating Scale

0	2	4	6	8	10
No Pain	A Little Pain	A Little More Pain	Even More Pain	A Whole Lot Of Pain	Worst Pain

Notes:

_____

_____

_____

_____

_____

_____

_____

Remember to check out the Release phases of body chemistry and stress biology action plans.

DAY 1 AFFIRMATION

Write it down. Say it out loud. Repeat often.

"I trust my body."

_____

_____

_____

_____

_____

_____

_____

_____

_____

_____

DAY 1 MINDSET MOJO

Food for thought. Try it.

Think of and speak of your pain in the past tense.

What does this bring up for you? Write about it. Free associate.

_____

_____

_____

_____

_____

_____

_____

_____

_____

_____

RELEASE – DAY 2

TODAY'S DATE: _____

Pick up to three of the following RELEASE activities:

(Go to the Exercise Index in the Resources section at the back of the book, Fix the Fire Damage, to help you find these activities.)

☐ Lie down and support your neck

☐ Lie down and support your low back

☐ Lie down and support your low back + hip

☐ Sleep position strategy +/or posture reset

☐ Sleep position strategy face up

☐ Sleep position strategy side lying

☐ Sleep position strategy belly face down

☐ Partial Bruegger's Relief positioning

☐ Pendulum passive release

☐ Seated to standing transition

☐ Hip rotator release against the wall

☐ Modified sphinx pose

☐ Hamstring stretch

RELEASE ACTIVITIES

RELEASE Activity #1: _____

Better? _____   Worse? _____   Same? _____

Other: _____

Notes: _____

_____

RELEASE Activity #2: _____

Better? _____   Worse? _____   Same? _____

Other: _____

Notes: _____

_____

RELEASE Activity #3: _____

Better? _____   Worse? _____   Same? _____

Other: _____

Notes: _____

_____

PAIN LOCATION:

Use this figure to color or shade-in the area of your pain however you like.

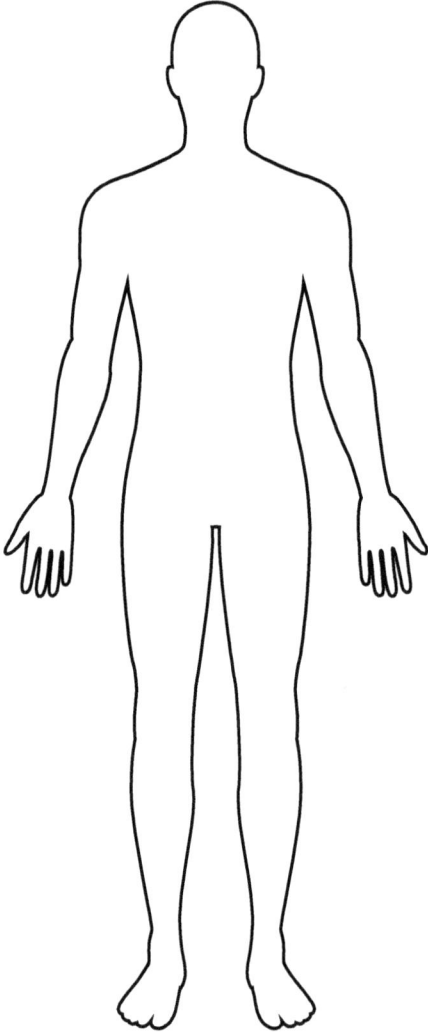

Quick Guide: Pain Locations

As seen in *The Everyday Pain Guide—Fix the Fire Damage*

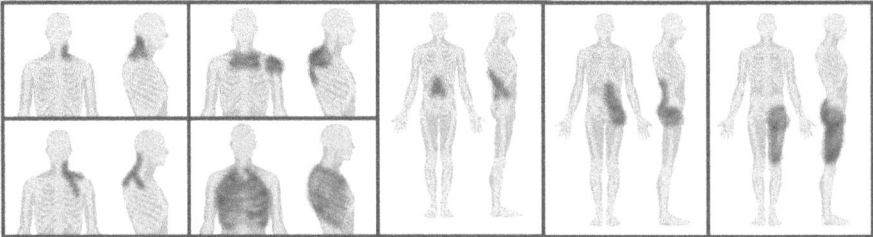

HOW MUCH PAIN TODAY?

Circle the face that best expresses your discomfort:

Wong-Baker FACES® Pain Rating Scale

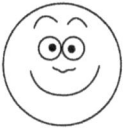 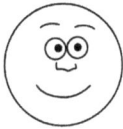 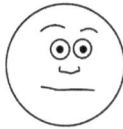 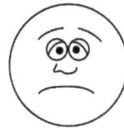 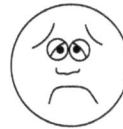 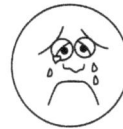

0	**2**	**4**	**6**	**8**	**10**
No Pain	A Little Pain	A Little More Pain	Even More Pain	A Whole Lot Of Pain	Worst Pain

Notes:

_____

_____

_____

_____

_____

_____

_____

Remember to check out the Release phases of body chemistry and stress biology action plans.

DAY 2 AFFIRMATION

Write it down. Say it out loud. Repeat often.

"My body is doing exactly what it's supposed to."

_____

_____

_____

_____

_____

_____

_____

_____

_____

_____

DAY 2 MINDSET MOJO

Food for thought. Try it.

Be kind to yourself!

What does this bring up for you? Write about it. Free associate.

_____

_____

_____

_____

_____

_____

_____

_____

_____

_____

_____

_____

_____

RELEASE – DAY 3

TODAY'S DATE: _____

Pick up to three of the following RELEASE activities:

(Go to the Exercise Index in the Resources section at the back of the book, Fix the Fire Damage, to help you find these activities.)

- ☐ Lie down and support your neck
- ☐ Lie down and support your low back
- ☐ Lie down and support your low back + hip
- ☐ Sleep position strategy +/or posture reset
- ☐ Sleep position strategy face up
- ☐ Sleep position strategy side lying
- ☐ Sleep position strategy belly face down
- ☐ Partial Bruegger's Relief positioning
- ☐ Pendulum passive release
- ☐ Seated to standing transition
- ☐ Hip rotator release against the wall
- ☐ Modified sphinx pose
- ☐ Hamstring stretch

RELEASE ACTIVITIES

RELEASE Activity #1: _____

Better? _____   Worse? _____   Same? _____

Other: _____

Notes: _____

_____

RELEASE Activity #2: _____

Better? _____   Worse? _____   Same? _____

Other: _____

Notes: _____

_____

RELEASE Activity #3: _____

Better? _____   Worse? _____   Same? _____

Other: _____

Notes: _____

_____

PAIN LOCATION:

Use this figure to color or shade-in the area of your pain however you like.

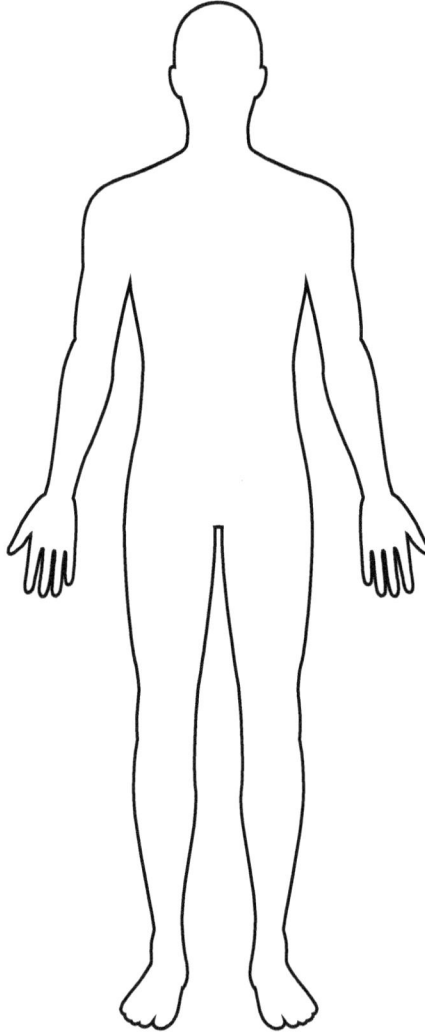

Quick Guide: Pain Locations

As seen in *The Everyday Pain Guide—Fix the Fire Damage*

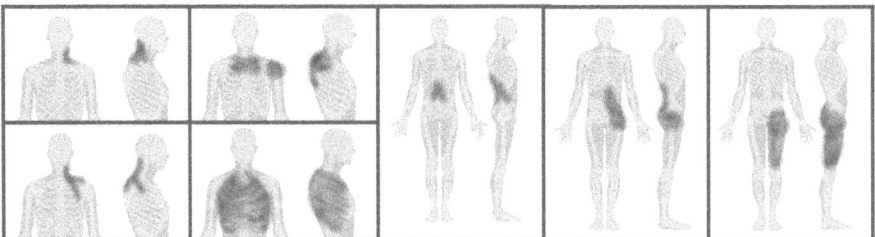

HOW MUCH PAIN TODAY?

Circle the face that best expresses your discomfort:

Wong-Baker FACES® Pain Rating Scale

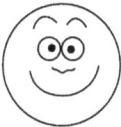 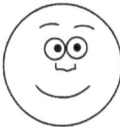 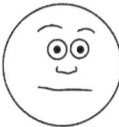 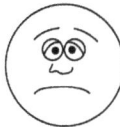 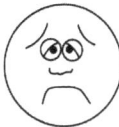 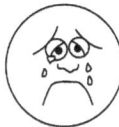

0	**2**	**4**	**6**	**8**	**10**
No Pain	A Little Pain	A Little More Pain	Even More Pain	A Whole Lot Of Pain	Worst Pain

Notes:

_____

_____

_____

_____

_____

_____

_____

Remember to check out the Release phases of body chemistry and stress biology action plans.

DAY 3 AFFIRMATION

Write it down. Say it out loud. Repeat often.

"I have a strong and resilient body."

_____

_____

_____

_____

_____

_____

_____

_____

_____

_____

DAY 3 MINDSET MOJO

Food for thought. Try it.

What happens when you listen to your pain?

What does this bring up for you? Write about it. Free associate.

_____

_____

_____

_____

_____

_____

_____

_____

_____

_____

TODAY'S DATE: _____

Pick up to three of the following RELEASE activities:

(Go to the Exercise Index in the Resources section at the back of the book, Fix the Fire Damage, to help you find these activities.)

- ☐ Lie down and support your neck

- ☐ Lie down and support your low back

- ☐ Lie down and support your low back + hip

- ☐ Sleep position strategy +/or posture reset

- ☐ Sleep position strategy face up

- ☐ Sleep position strategy side lying

- ☐ Sleep position strategy belly face down

- ☐ Partial Bruegger's Relief positioning

- ☐ Pendulum passive release

- ☐ Seated to standing transition

- ☐ Hip rotator release against the wall

- ☐ Modified sphinx pose

- ☐ Hamstring stretch

RELEASE ACTIVITIES

RELEASE Activity #1: _____

Better? _____   Worse? _____   Same? _____

Other:_____

Notes:_____

_____

RELEASE Activity #2: _____

Better? _____   Worse? _____   Same? _____

Other:_____

Notes:_____

_____

RELEASE Activity #3: _____

Better? _____   Worse? _____   Same? _____

Other:_____

Notes:_____

_____

PAIN LOCATION:

Use this figure to color or shade-in the area of your pain however you like.

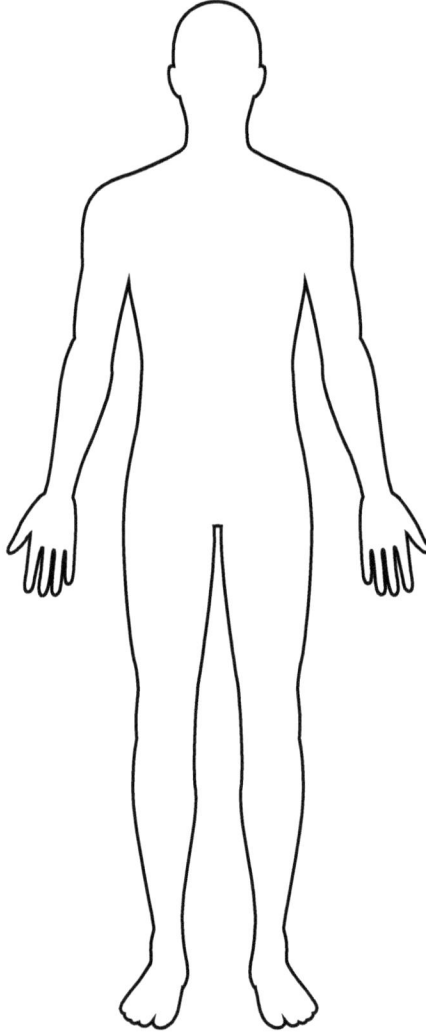

Quick Guide: Pain Locations

As seen in *The Everyday Pain Guide—Fix the Fire Damage*

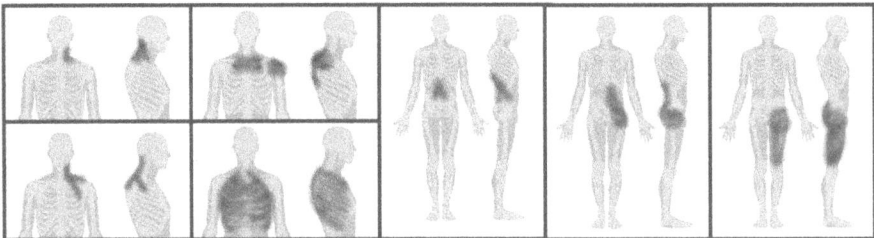

HOW MUCH PAIN TODAY?

Circle the face that best expresses your discomfort:

Wong-Baker FACES® Pain Rating Scale

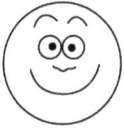 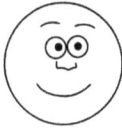 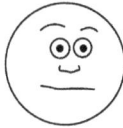 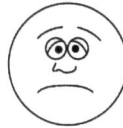 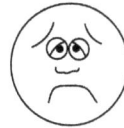 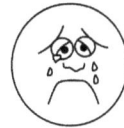

0	2	4	6	8	10
No Pain	A Little Pain	A Little More Pain	Even More Pain	A Whole Lot Of Pain	Worst Pain

Notes:

_____

_____

_____

_____

_____

_____

_____

Remember to check out the Release phases of body chemistry and stress biology action plans.

DAY 4 AFFIRMATION

Write it down. Say it out loud. Repeat often.

"My body knows just what to do."

_____

_____

_____

_____

_____

_____

_____

_____

_____

_____

DAY 4 MINDSET MOJO

Food for thought. Try it.

You did nothing wrong.

What does this bring up for you? Write about it. Free associate.

_____

_____

_____

_____

_____

_____

_____

_____

_____

_____

_____

_____

RELEASE – DAY 5

TODAY'S DATE: _____

Pick up to three of the following RELEASE activities:

(Go to the Exercise Index in the Resources section at the back of the book, Fix the Fire Damage, to help you find these activities.)

- ☐ Lie down and support your neck

- ☐ Lie down and support your low back

- ☐ Lie down and support your low back + hip

- ☐ Sleep position strategy +/or posture reset

- ☐ Sleep position strategy face up

- ☐ Sleep position strategy side lying

- ☐ Sleep position strategy belly face down

- ☐ Partial Bruegger's Relief positioning

- ☐ Pendulum passive release

- ☐ Seated to standing transition

- ☐ Hip rotator release against the wall

- ☐ Modified sphinx pose

- ☐ Hamstring stretch

RELEASE ACTIVITIES

RELEASE Activity #1: _____

Better? _____   Worse? _____   Same? _____

Other: _____

Notes: _____

_____

RELEASE Activity #2: _____

Better? _____   Worse? _____   Same? _____

Other: _____

Notes: _____

_____

RELEASE Activity #3: _____

Better? _____   Worse? _____   Same? _____

Other: _____

Notes: _____

_____

PAIN LOCATION:

Use this figure to color or shade-in the area of your pain however you like.

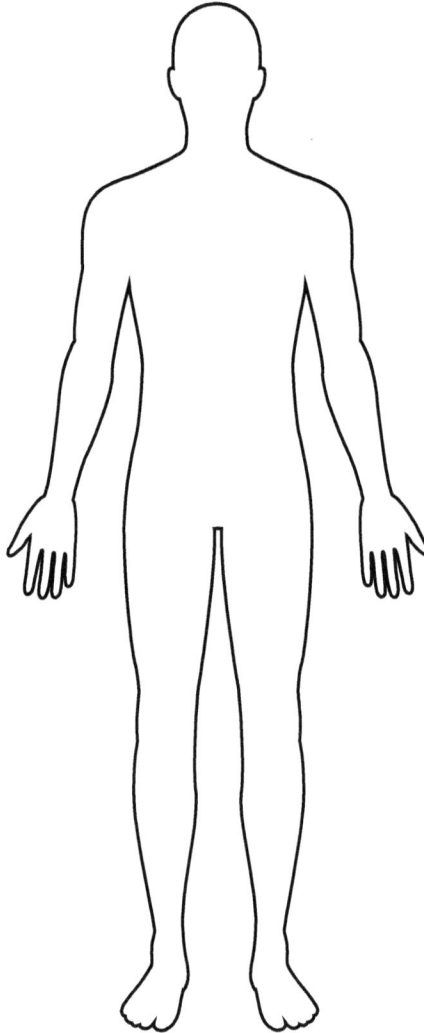

Quick Guide: Pain Locations

As seen in *The Everyday Pain Guide—Fix the Fire Damage*

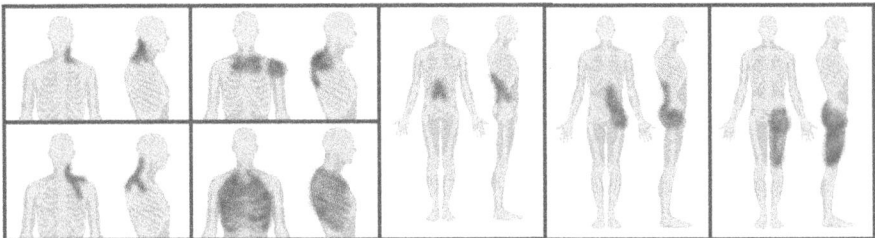

HOW MUCH PAIN TODAY?

Circle the face that best expresses your discomfort:

Wong-Baker FACES® Pain Rating Scale

0	2	4	6	8	10
No Pain	A Little Pain	A Little More Pain	Even More Pain	A Whole Lot Of Pain	Worst Pain

Notes:

_____

_____

_____

_____

_____

_____

_____

_____

Remember to check out the Release phases of body chemistry and stress biology action plans.

DAY 5 AFFIRMATION

Write it down. Say it out loud. Repeat often.

"My pain is a sensible message and I'm listening."

_____

_____

_____

_____

_____

_____

_____

_____

_____

_____

DAY 5 MINDSET MOJO

Food for thought. Try it.

You are doing your best and that is enough.

What does this bring up for you? Write about it. Free associate.

_____

_____

_____

_____

_____

_____

_____

_____

_____

_____

_____

RELEASE - DAY 6

TODAY'S DATE: _____

Pick up to three of the following RELEASE activities:

(Go to the Exercise Index in the Resources section at the back of the book, Fix the Fire Damage, to help you find these activities.)

- ☐ Lie down and support your neck

- ☐ Lie down and support your low back

- ☐ Lie down and support your low back + hip

- ☐ Sleep position strategy +/or posture reset

- ☐ Sleep position strategy face up

- ☐ Sleep position strategy side lying

- ☐ Sleep position strategy belly face down

- ☐ Partial Bruegger's Relief positioning

- ☐ Pendulum passive release

- ☐ Seated to standing transition

- ☐ Hip rotator release against the wall

- ☐ Modified sphinx pose

- ☐ Hamstring stretch

RELEASE ACTIVITIES

RELEASE Activity #1: _____

Better? _____   Worse? _____   Same? _____

Other: _____

Notes: _____

_____

RELEASE Activity #2: _____

Better? _____   Worse? _____   Same? _____

Other: _____

Notes: _____

_____

RELEASE Activity #3: _____

Better? _____   Worse? _____   Same? _____

Other: _____

Notes: _____

_____

PAIN LOCATION:

Use this figure to color or shade-in the area of your pain however you like.

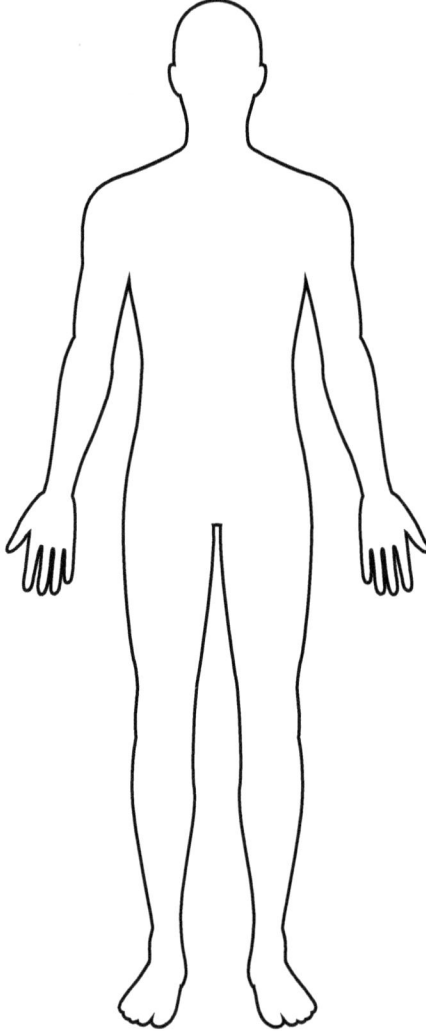

Quick Guide: Pain Locations

As seen in *The Everyday Pain Guide—Fix the Fire Damage*

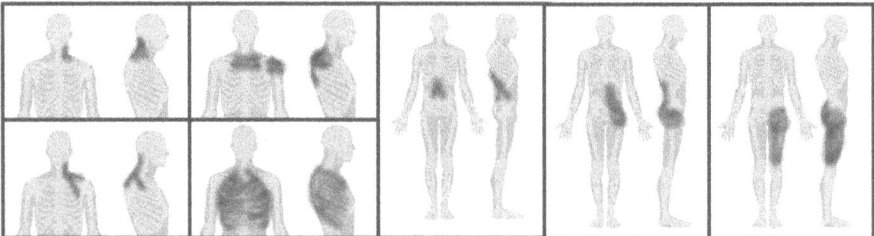

HOW MUCH PAIN TODAY?

Circle the face that best expresses your discomfort:

Wong-Baker FACES® Pain Rating Scale

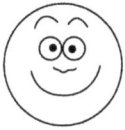 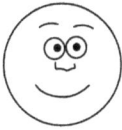 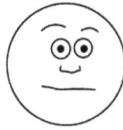 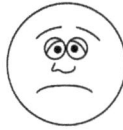 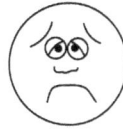 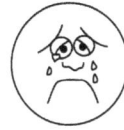

0	**2**	**4**	**6**	**8**	**10**
No Pain	A Little Pain	A Little More Pain	Even More Pain	A Whole Lot Of Pain	Worst Pain

Notes:

_____

_____

_____

_____

_____

_____

_____

Remember to check out the Release phases of body chemistry and stress biology action plans.

DAY 6 AFFIRMATION

Write it down. Say it out loud. Repeat often.

"My body is telling me something important about how to move forward into better health."

_____

_____

_____

_____

_____

_____

_____

_____

_____

DAY 6 MINDSET MOJO

Food for thought. Try it.

Breathe.

What does this bring up for you? Write about it. Free associate.

_____

_____

_____

_____

_____

_____

_____

_____

_____

_____

RELEASE – DAY 7

TODAY'S DATE: _____

Pick up to three of the following RELEASE activities:

(Go to the Exercise Index in the Resources section at the back of the book, Fix the Fire Damage, to help you find these activities.)

☐ Lie down and support your neck

☐ Lie down and support your low back

☐ Lie down and support your low back + hip

☐ Sleep position strategy +/or posture reset

☐ Sleep position strategy face up

☐ Sleep position strategy side lying

☐ Sleep position strategy belly face down

☐ Partial Bruegger's Relief positioning

☐ Pendulum passive release

☐ Seated to standing transition

☐ Hip rotator release against the wall

☐ Modified sphinx pose

☐ Hamstring stretch

RELEASE ACTIVITIES

RELEASE Activity #1: _____

Better? _____   Worse? _____   Same? _____

Other: _____

Notes: _____

_____

RELEASE Activity #2: _____

Better? _____   Worse? _____   Same? _____

Other: _____

Notes: _____

_____

RELEASE Activity #3: _____

Better? _____   Worse? _____   Same? _____

Other: _____

Notes: _____

_____

PAIN LOCATION:

Use this figure to color or shade-in the area of your pain however you like.

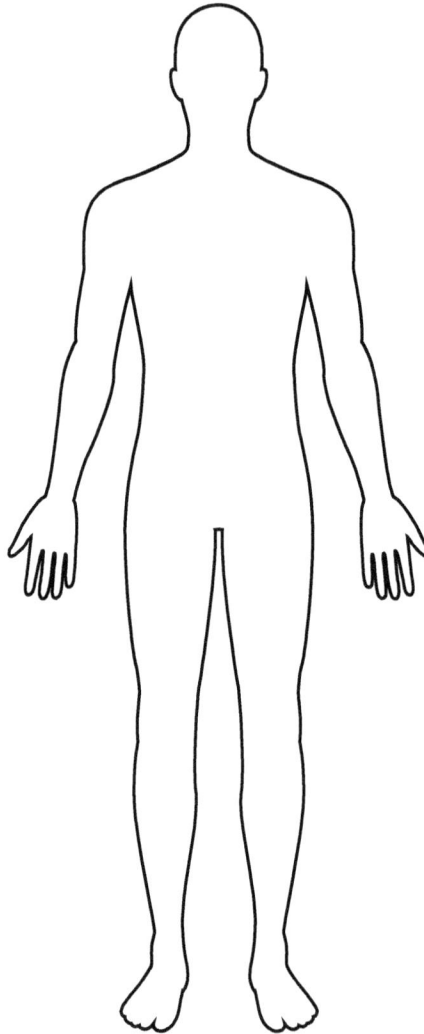

Quick Guide: Pain Locations

As seen in *The Everyday Pain Guide—Fix the Fire Damage*

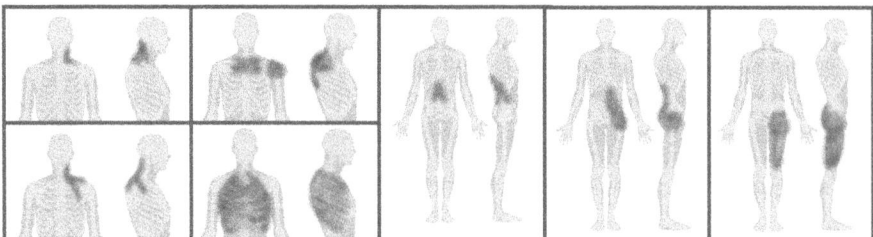

HOW MUCH PAIN TODAY?

Circle the face that best expresses your discomfort:

Wong-Baker FACES® Pain Rating Scale

0	2	4	6	8	10
No Pain	A Little Pain	A Little More Pain	Even More Pain	A Whole Lot Of Pain	Worst Pain

Notes:

_____

_____

_____

_____

_____

_____

_____

Remember to check out the Release phases of body chemistry and stress biology action plans.

DAY 7 AFFIRMATION

Write it down. Say it out loud. Repeat often.

"My body is watching out for me and all is well."

_____

_____

_____

_____

_____

_____

_____

_____

_____

_____

_____

DAY 7 MINDSET MOJO

Food for thought. Try it.

You are not alone.

What does this bring up for you? Write about it. Free associate.

_____

_____

_____

_____

_____

_____

_____

_____

_____

_____

Have you completed the Release phase of action?

Q: Is your pain making you change your daytime routine or sleeping habits?

Circle one: Yes / No

Details:_____

_____

_____

_____

_____

Q: Do you find yourself unable to carry on a regular day of tasks without feeling some of the pain?

Circle one: Yes / No

Details:_____

_____

_____

_____

_____

Q: Do you feel fine in the morning, but your pain gets worse as the day goes on?

Circle one: Yes / No

Details:_____

_____

_____

_____

_____

If you answered YES to any of these questions, then you do need to continue with your Release activities even if you are ready to move forward. Take it slow. Review and repeat your last 7 days.

Are you ready for the next phase of action - Retrain?

Q: Do you still feel the pain here and there but you're able to complete your daily tasks uninterrupted without special modifications?

Circle one: Yes / No

Details:_____

_____

_____

_____

_____

_____

_____

_____

_____

_____

_____

Q: Do you still feel some pain in bed at night, but no longer have to think too much about your positioning and pillow support to fall asleep?

Circle one: Yes / No

Details:_____

_____

_____

_____

_____

_____

_____

_____

If you answered YES to one or both of these questions, then you are ready to try the Retrain activities.

Consider revisiting the Release activities even as you dip your toe into the Retrain phase. It's natural to have days when it feels like you've taken a step or two backwards.

"No matter how
hard the past,
you can always
begin again."

—Buddha Gautama

My *Retrain* Action Steps

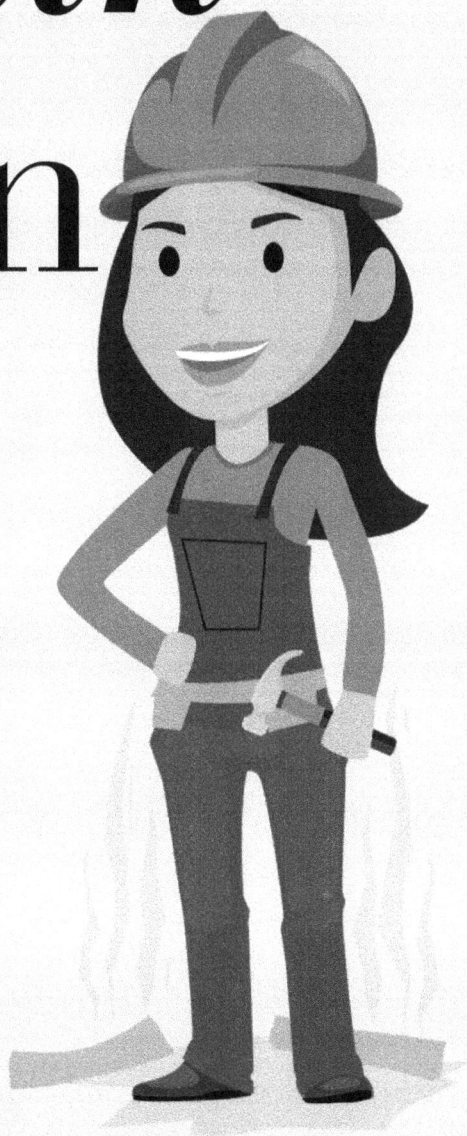

THE CHECK IN

How are you feeling?

TODAY'S DATE: _____

PAIN LOCATION:
(circle one)

Neck   Neck/Shoulder   Shoulder/Upper Back   Mid Back/Torso/Ribs

Low Back   Low Back/Hip   Hip/Buttock/Thigh

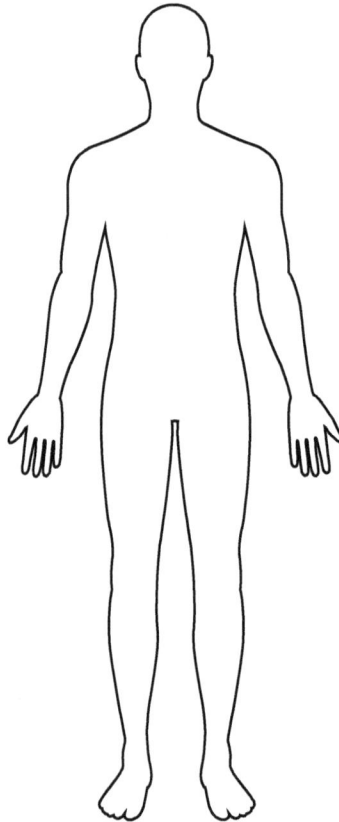

Use this figure to color or shade-in the area of your pain however you like.

HOW MUCH PAIN TODAY?

Circle the face below that best expresses your discomfort:

Wong-Baker FACES® Pain Rating Scale

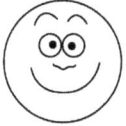 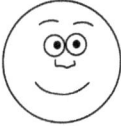 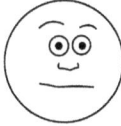 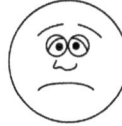 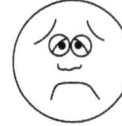 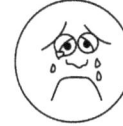

0	**2**	**4**	**6**	**8**	**10**
No Pain	A Little Pain	A Little More Pain	Even More Pain	A Whole Lot Of Pain	Worst Pain

- If you circled #4, consider continuing with your Release actions while proceeding.
- If you circled #6 or higher, please return to Release for at least another week before proceeding.

Notes:

_____

_____

_____

_____

_____

_____

My pain feels:
(circle all that apply)

Sharp   Stabbing   Achy   Tingly   Throbbing

Grabbing   Tightness   Pinching

Other/More Details: _____

_____

_____

_____

_____

When do I notice it the *most*?
(circle all that apply)

Sitting   Standing still   Walking   Getting up from sitting

Lying on my back   Lying on my belly   Lying on my RIGHT side

Lying on my LEFT side   Driving the car   Mornings

Before bed   Middle of the night

Other/More Details: _____

_____

_____

_____

When do I notice it *less*?
(circle all that apply)

Sitting   Standing still   Walking   Getting up from sitting

Lying on my back   Lying on my belly   Lying on my RIGHT side

Lying on my LEFT side   Driving the car   Mornings

Before bed   Middle of the night

Other/More Details: _____

_____

_____

_____

_____

Medication used:
(circle all that apply)

Ibuprofen (Motrin/Advil)   Naproxen (Aleve)   Acetaminophen (Tylenol)

Other/Prescription: _____

_____

How much? _____

_____

☐ Some Relief?   ☐ Total Relief?   ☐ No Relief?

RETRAIN!

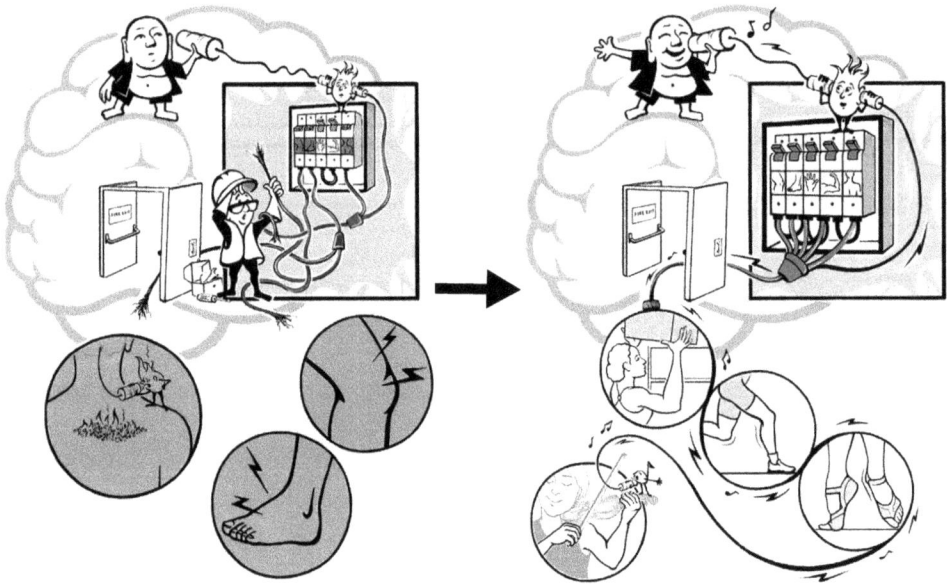

Restore communication. To avoid falling into a neurological rut of dysfunctional adaptation, retraining is needed to reprogram parts of your brain and nervous system that communicate with the vulnerable area in pain. To retrain is to resume nurturing those connections.

Q: *What* are you retraining?

A: **Your proprioception (the position-sensing and movement-coordinating part of the brain)**

Q: *How* are you retraining your proprioception?

A: **With strategic isometric activity**

NEXT STEPS:

1. Return to the action plan for your pain location in The *Everyday Pain Guide – Fix the Fire Damage.*

2. This time try all **Retrain** activities associated with your pain location.

3. Pick up to three **Retrain** activities for daily use and record your progress in the following pages…

The steps in this Retrain phase of the Body Mechanics Action Plans will help you return to motion safely by reactivating the injured or stressed areas. You'll be given specific strategies focusing on isometric exercise (activation without movement) with safe and subtle positioning to help the connections between your brain and the injured or stressed area switch back "on" as soon as possible after inflammation flares.

Retrain action steps may not be pain-free to implement, but they will help you safely continue the repair process while restoring the brain-body connection.

It is possible to be in the middle of the Retrain phase of your repair process yet still need to occasionally revisit earlier Release action steps for the calming and cooling strategies designed to provide relief, so don't close the book on that phase completely just yet!

Notes:

_____

_____

_____

_____

_____

_____

_____

_____

_____

_____

_____

_____

_____

_____

Retrain
Activities

Week One

RETRAIN – DAY 1

TODAY'S DATE: _____

Pick up to three of the following RETRAIN activities:

(Go to the Exercise Index in the Resources section at the back of the book, *Fix the Fire Damage*, to help you find these activities.)

- [ ] Posterior isometrics – neutral
- [ ] Posterior isometrics – at 45 deg.
- [ ] Shoulder shrug isometric
- [ ] Eagle arms pose
- [ ] Reach for the ceiling
- [ ] Wall plank
- [ ] Arm reach isometric
- [ ] External shoulder rotation isometric
- [ ] Triceps extension pulldown isometric
- [ ] Modified sphinx pose
- [ ] Shoulder shrug isometric – mid

- [ ] Bent over fly isometric – torso supported
- [ ] Inner thigh isometrics
- [ ] Superman isometrics with lower back and hip focus
- [ ] Clamshell isometric
- [ ] Hamstring stretch – active
- [ ] Reverse roman chair – isometric
- [ ] Squats with ball against wall – isometric
- [ ] Bridge marching
- [ ] Upward dog
- [ ] Ball-Wall hip stability isometric

RETRAIN ACTIVITIES

RETRAIN Activity #1: _____

Better? _____   Worse? _____   Same? _____

Other: _____

Notes: _____

_____

RETRAIN Activity #2: _____

Better? _____   Worse? _____   Same? _____

Other: _____

Notes: _____

_____

RETRAIN Activity #3: _____

Better? _____   Worse? _____   Same? _____

Other: _____

Notes: _____

_____

PAIN LOCATION:

Use this figure to color or shade-in the area of your pain however you like.

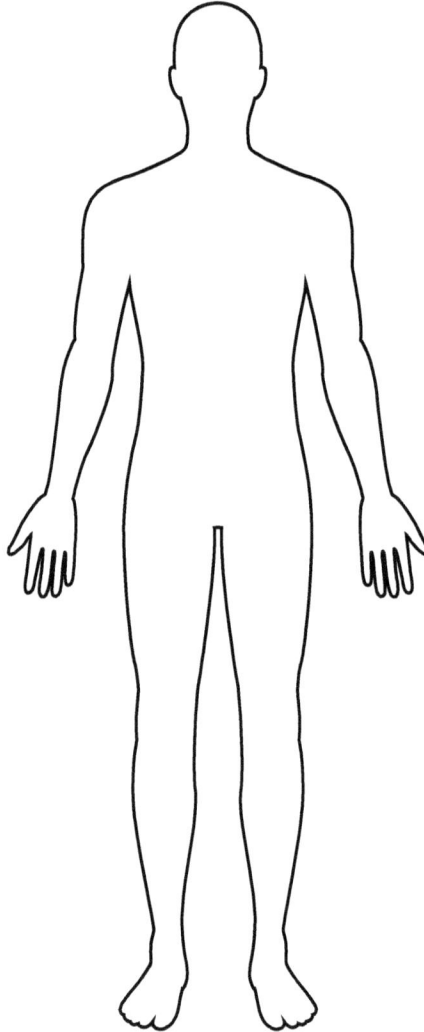

Quick Guide: Pain Locations

As seen in *The Everyday Pain Guide—Fix the Fire Damage*

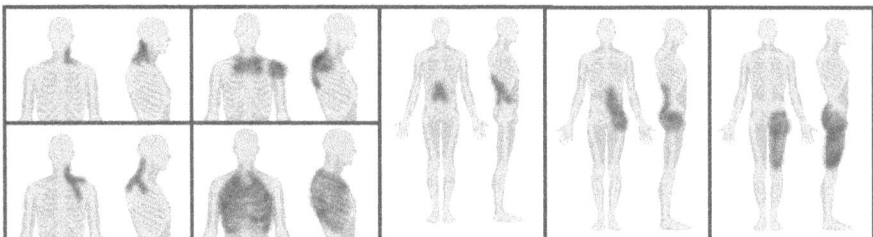

HOW MUCH PAIN TODAY?

Circle the face that best expresses your discomfort:

Wong-Baker FACES® Pain Rating Scale

0	2	4	6	8	10
No Pain	A Little Pain	A Little More Pain	Even More Pain	A Whole Lot Of Pain	Worst Pain

Notes:

_____

_____

_____

_____

_____

_____

_____

Remember to check out the Retrain phases of body chemistry and stress biology action plans.

RETRAIN – DAY 2

TODAY'S DATE: _____

Pick up to three of the following RETRAIN activities:

(Go to the Exercise Index in the Resources section at the back of the book, *Fix the Fire Damage*, to help you find these activities.)

☐ Posterior isometrics – neutral

☐ Posterior isometrics – at 45 deg.

☐ Shoulder shrug isometric

☐ Eagle arms pose

☐ Reach for the ceiling

☐ Wall plank

☐ Arm reach isometric

☐ External shoulder rotation isometric

☐ Triceps extension pulldown isometric

☐ Modified sphinx pose

☐ Shoulder shrug isometric – mid

☐ Bent over fly isometric – torso supported

☐ Inner thigh isometrics

☐ Superman isometrics with lower back and hip focus

☐ Clamshell isometric

☐ Hamstring stretch – active

☐ Reverse roman chair – isometric

☐ Squats with ball against wall – isometric

☐ Bridge marching

☐ Upward dog

☐ Ball-Wall hip stability isometric

RETRAIN ACTIVITIES

RETRAIN Activity #1: _____

Better? _____   Worse? _____   Same? _____

Other: _____

Notes: _____

_____

RETRAIN Activity #2: _____

Better? _____   Worse? _____   Same? _____

Other: _____

Notes: _____

_____

RETRAIN Activity #3: _____

Better? _____   Worse? _____   Same? _____

Other: _____

Notes: _____

_____

PAIN LOCATION:

Use this figure to color or shade-in the area of your pain however you like.

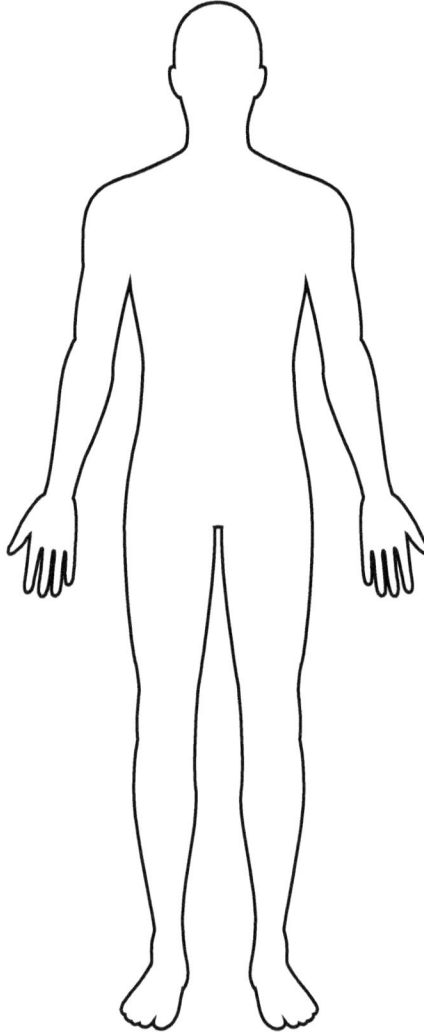

Quick Guide: Pain Locations

As seen in *The Everyday Pain Guide—Fix the Fire Damage*

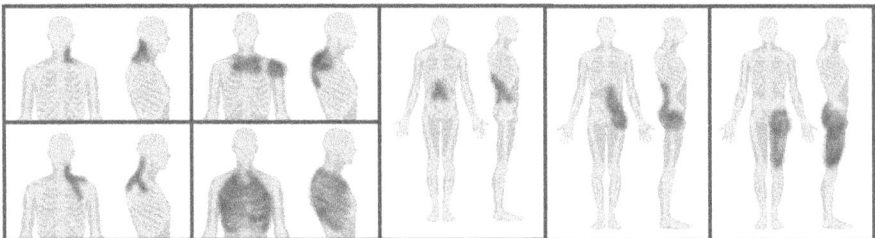

HOW MUCH PAIN TODAY?

Circle the face that best expresses your discomfort:

Wong-Baker FACES® Pain Rating Scale

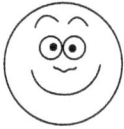 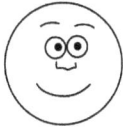 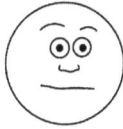 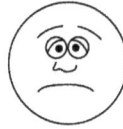 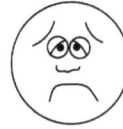 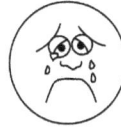

0	2	4	6	8	10
No Pain	A Little Pain	A Little More Pain	Even More Pain	A Whole Lot Of Pain	Worst Pain

Notes:

_____

_____

_____

_____

_____

_____

_____

Remember to check out the Retrain phases of body chemistry and stress biology action plans.

TODAY'S DATE: _____

Pick up to three of the following RETRAIN activities:

(Go to the Exercise Index in the Resources section at the back of the book, *Fix the Fire Damage*, to help you find these activities.)

☐ Posterior isometrics – neutral

☐ Bent over fly isometric – torso supported

☐ Posterior isometrics – at 45 deg.

☐ Inner thigh isometrics

☐ Shoulder shrug isometric

☐ Superman isometrics with lower back and hip focus

☐ Eagle arms pose

☐ Clamshell isometric

☐ Reach for the ceiling

☐ Hamstring stretch – active

☐ Wall plank

☐ Reverse roman chair – isometric

☐ Arm reach isometric

☐ Squats with ball against wall – isometric

☐ External shoulder rotation isometric

☐ Bridge marching

☐ Triceps extension pulldown isometric

☐ Upward dog

☐ Modified sphinx pose

☐ Ball-Wall hip stability isometric

☐ Shoulder shrug isometric – mid

RETRAIN ACTIVITIES

RETRAIN Activity #1: _____

Better? _____   Worse? _____   Same? _____

Other: _____

Notes: _____

_____

RETRAIN Activity #2: _____

Better? _____   Worse? _____   Same? _____

Other: _____

Notes: _____

_____

RETRAIN Activity #3: _____

Better? _____   Worse? _____   Same? _____

Other: _____

Notes: _____

_____

PAIN LOCATION:

Use this figure to color or shade-in the area of your pain however you like.

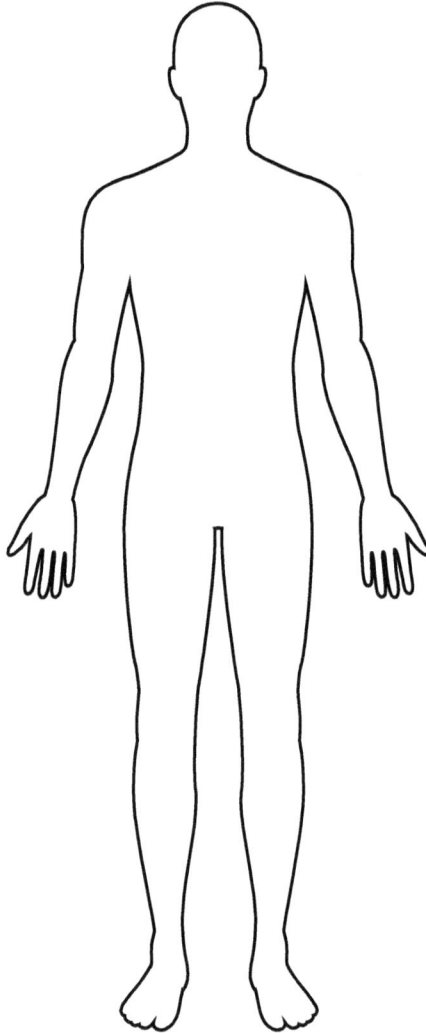

Quick Guide: Pain Locations

As seen in *The Everyday Pain Guide—Fix the Fire Damage*

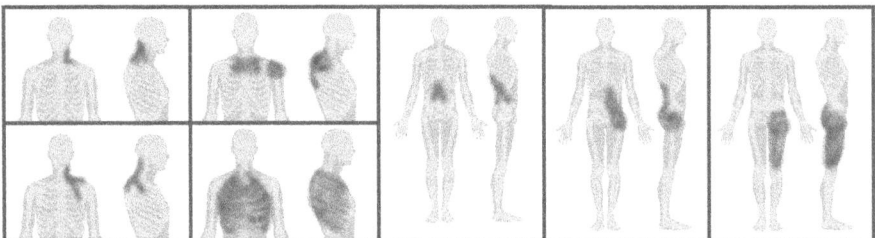

HOW MUCH PAIN TODAY?

Circle the face that best expresses your discomfort:

Wong-Baker FACES® Pain Rating Scale

0	2	4	6	8	10
No Pain	A Little Pain	A Little More Pain	Even More Pain	A Whole Lot Of Pain	Worst Pain

Notes:

_____

_____

_____

_____

_____

_____

_____

Remember to check out the Retrain phases of body chemistry and stress biology action plans.

TODAY'S DATE: _____

Pick up to three of the following RETRAIN activities:

(Go to the Exercise Index in the Resources section at the back of the book, *Fix the Fire Damage*, to help you find these activities.)

- ☐ Posterior isometrics – neutral
- ☐ Posterior isometrics – at 45 deg.
- ☐ Shoulder shrug isometric
- ☐ Eagle arms pose
- ☐ Reach for the ceiling
- ☐ Wall plank
- ☐ Arm reach isometric
- ☐ External shoulder rotation isometric
- ☐ Triceps extension pulldown isometric
- ☐ Modified sphinx pose
- ☐ Shoulder shrug isometric – mid

- ☐ Bent over fly isometric – torso supported
- ☐ Inner thigh isometrics
- ☐ Superman isometrics with lower back and hip focus
- ☐ Clamshell isometric
- ☐ Hamstring stretch – active
- ☐ Reverse roman chair – isometric
- ☐ Squats with ball against wall – isometric
- ☐ Bridge marching
- ☐ Upward dog
- ☐ Ball-Wall hip stability isometric

RETRAIN ACTIVITIES

RETRAIN Activity #1: _____

Better? _____   Worse? _____   Same? _____

Other: _____

Notes: _____

_____

RETRAIN Activity #2: _____

Better? _____   Worse? _____   Same? _____

Other: _____

Notes: _____

_____

RETRAIN Activity #3: _____

Better? _____   Worse? _____   Same? _____

Other: _____

Notes: _____

_____

PAIN LOCATION:

Use this figure to color or shade-in the area of your pain however you like.

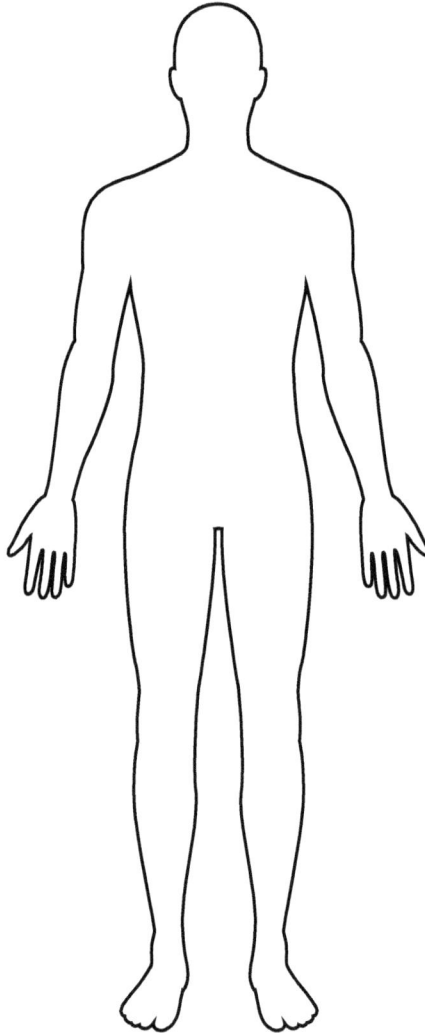

Quick Guide: Pain Locations

As seen in *The Everyday Pain Guide—Fix the Fire Damage*

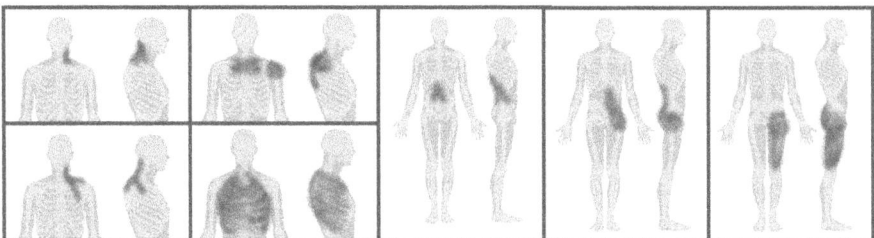

HOW MUCH PAIN TODAY?

Circle the face that best expresses your discomfort:

Wong-Baker FACES® Pain Rating Scale

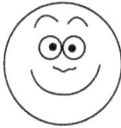 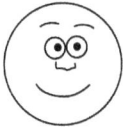 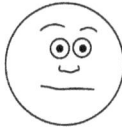 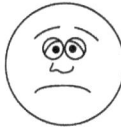 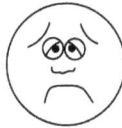 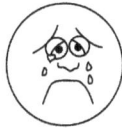

0	2	4	6	8	10
No Pain	A Little Pain	A Little More Pain	Even More Pain	A Whole Lot Of Pain	Worst Pain

Notes:

_____

_____

_____

_____

_____

_____

_____

_____

Remember to check out the Retrain phases of body chemistry and stress biology action plans.

TODAY'S DATE: _____

Pick up to three of the following RETRAIN activities:

(Go to the Exercise Index in the Resources section at the back of the book, *Fix the Fire Damage*, to help you find these activities.)

☐ Posterior isometrics – neutral

☐ Posterior isometrics – at 45 deg.

☐ Shoulder shrug isometric

☐ Eagle arms pose

☐ Reach for the ceiling

☐ Wall plank

☐ Arm reach isometric

☐ External shoulder rotation isometric

☐ Triceps extension pulldown isometric

☐ Modified sphinx pose

☐ Shoulder shrug isometric – mid

☐ Bent over fly isometric – torso supported

☐ Inner thigh isometrics

☐ Superman isometrics with lower back and hip focus

☐ Clamshell isometric

☐ Hamstring stretch – active

☐ Reverse roman chair – isometric

☐ Squats with ball against wall – isometric

☐ Bridge marching

☐ Upward dog

☐ Ball-Wall hip stability isometric

RETRAIN ACTIVITIES

RETRAIN Activity #1: _____

Better? _____   Worse? _____   Same? _____

Other: _____

Notes: _____

_____

RETRAIN Activity #2: _____

Better? _____   Worse? _____   Same? _____

Other: _____

Notes: _____

_____

RETRAIN Activity #3: _____

Better? _____   Worse? _____   Same? _____

Other: _____

Notes: _____

_____

PAIN LOCATION:

Use this figure to color or shade-in the area of your pain however you like.

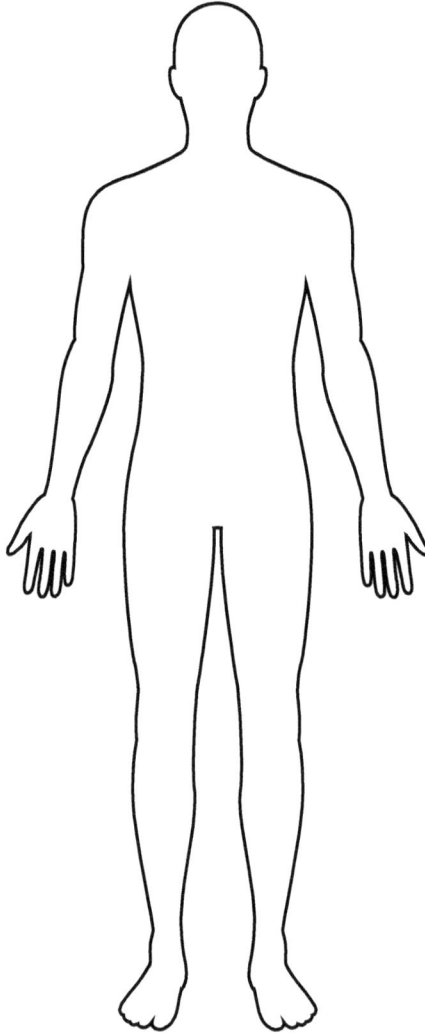

Quick Guide: Pain Locations

As seen in *The Everyday Pain Guide—Fix the Fire Damage*

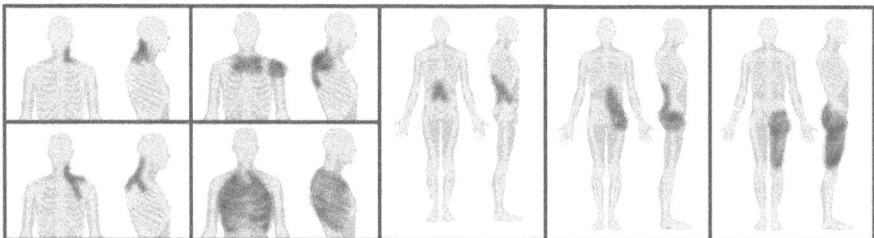

HOW MUCH PAIN TODAY?

Circle the face that best expresses your discomfort:

Wong-Baker FACES® Pain Rating Scale

0	2	4	6	8	10
No Pain	A Little Pain	A Little More Pain	Even More Pain	A Whole Lot Of Pain	Worst Pain

Notes:

_____

_____

_____

_____

_____

_____

_____

_____

Remember to check out the Retrain phases of body chemistry and stress biology action plans.

RETRAIN – DAY 6

TODAY'S DATE: _____

Pick up to three of the following RETRAIN activities:

(Go to the Exercise Index in the Resources section at the back of the book, Fix the Fire Damage, to help you find these activities.)

☐ Posterior isometrics – neutral

☐ Posterior isometrics – at 45 deg.

☐ Shoulder shrug isometric

☐ Eagle arms pose

☐ Reach for the ceiling

☐ Wall plank

☐ Arm reach isometric

☐ External shoulder rotation isometric

☐ Triceps extension pulldown isometric

☐ Modified sphinx pose

☐ Shoulder shrug isometric – mid

☐ Bent over fly isometric – torso supported

☐ Inner thigh isometrics

☐ Superman isometrics with lower back and hip focus

☐ Clamshell isometric

☐ Hamstring stretch – active

☐ Reverse roman chair – isometric

☐ Squats with ball against wall – isometric

☐ Bridge marching

☐ Upward dog

☐ Ball-Wall hip stability isometric

RETRAIN ACTIVITIES

RETRAIN Activity #1: _____

Better? _____   Worse? _____   Same? _____

Other: _____

Notes: _____

_____

RETRAIN Activity #2: _____

Better? _____   Worse? _____   Same? _____

Other: _____

Notes: _____

_____

RETRAIN Activity #3: _____

Better? _____   Worse? _____   Same? _____

Other: _____

Notes: _____

_____

PAIN LOCATION:

Use this figure to color or shade-in the area of your pain however you like.

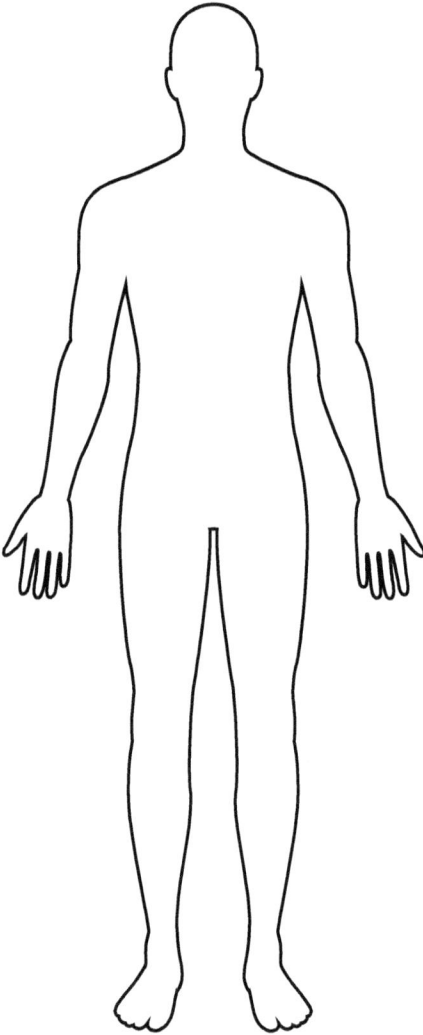

Quick Guide: Pain Locations

As seen in *The Everyday Pain Guide—Fix the Fire Damage*

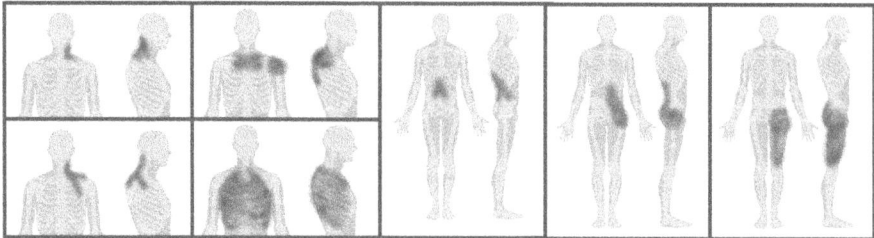

HOW MUCH PAIN TODAY?

Circle the face that best expresses your discomfort:

Wong-Baker FACES® Pain Rating Scale

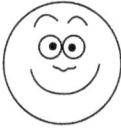 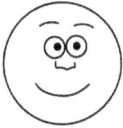 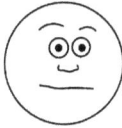 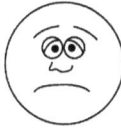 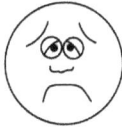 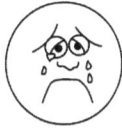

0	2	4	6	8	10
No Pain	A Little Pain	A Little More Pain	Even More Pain	A Whole Lot Of Pain	Worst Pain

Notes:

_____

_____

_____

_____

_____

_____

_____

_____

Remember to check out the Retrain phases of body chemistry and stress biology action plans.

RETRAIN – DAY 7

TODAY'S DATE: _____

Pick up to three of the following RETRAIN activities:

(Go to the Exercise Index in the Resources section at the back of the book, *Fix the Fire Damage*, to help you find these activities.)

☐ Posterior isometrics – neutral

☐ Bent over fly isometric – torso supported

☐ Posterior isometrics – at 45 deg.

☐ Inner thigh isometrics

☐ Shoulder shrug isometric

☐ Superman isometrics with lower back and hip focus

☐ Eagle arms pose

☐ Clamshell isometric

☐ Reach for the ceiling

☐ Hamstring stretch – active

☐ Wall plank

☐ Reverse roman chair – isometric

☐ Arm reach isometric

☐ Squats with ball against wall – isometric

☐ External shoulder rotation isometric

☐ Bridge marching

☐ Triceps extension pulldown isometric

☐ Upward dog

☐ Modified sphinx pose

☐ Ball-Wall hip stability isometric

☐ Shoulder shrug isometric – mid

RETRAIN ACTIVITIES

RETRAIN Activity #1: _____

Better? _____   Worse? _____   Same? _____

Other: _____

Notes: _____

_____

RETRAIN Activity #2: _____

Better? _____   Worse? _____   Same? _____

Other: _____

Notes: _____

_____

RETRAIN Activity #3: _____

Better? _____   Worse? _____   Same? _____

Other: _____

Notes: _____

_____

PAIN LOCATION:

Use this figure to color or shade-in the area of your pain however you like.

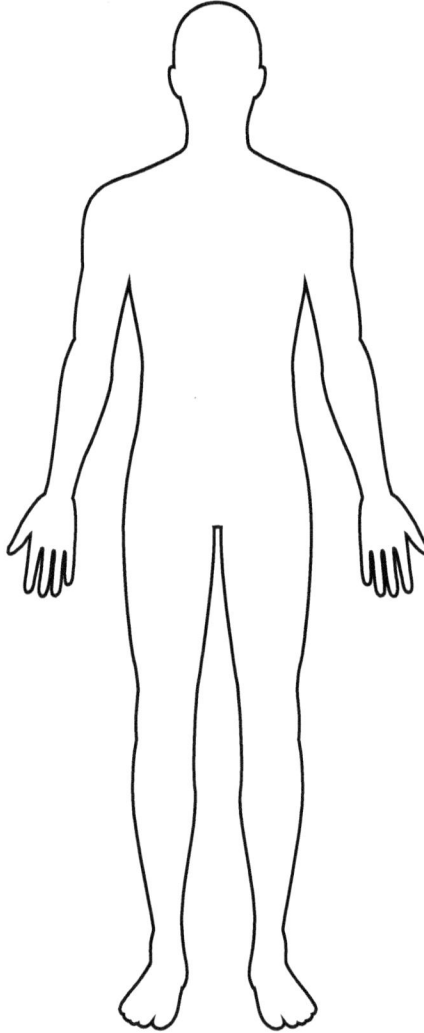

Quick Guide: Pain Locations

As seen in *The Everyday Pain Guide—Fix the Fire Damage*

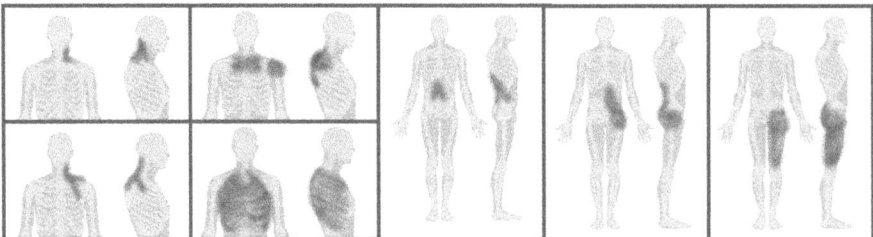

HOW MUCH PAIN TODAY?

Circle the face that best expresses your discomfort:

Wong-Baker FACES® Pain Rating Scale

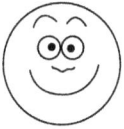 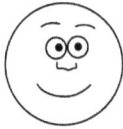 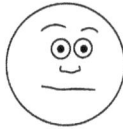 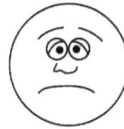 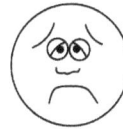 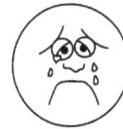

0	2	4	6	8	10
No Pain	A Little Pain	A Little More Pain	Even More Pain	A Whole Lot Of Pain	Worst Pain

Notes:

_____

_____

_____

_____

_____

_____

_____

Remember to check out the Retrain phases of body chemistry and stress biology action plans.

Notes:

_____

_____

_____

_____

_____

_____

_____

_____

_____

_____

_____

_____

_____

_____

_____

Retrain
Activities

Week Two

RETRAIN – DAY 1

TODAY'S DATE: _____

Pick up to three of the following RETRAIN activities:

(Go to the Exercise Index in the Resources section at the back of the book, *Fix the Fire Damage*, to help you find these activities.)

☐ Posterior isometrics – neutral

☐ Posterior isometrics – at 45 deg.

☐ Shoulder shrug isometric

☐ Eagle arms pose

☐ Reach for the ceiling

☐ Wall plank

☐ Arm reach isometric

☐ External shoulder rotation isometric

☐ Triceps extension pulldown isometric

☐ Modified sphinx pose

☐ Shoulder shrug isometric – mid

☐ Bent over fly isometric – torso supported

☐ Inner thigh isometrics

☐ Superman isometrics with lower back and hip focus

☐ Clamshell isometric

☐ Hamstring stretch – active

☐ Reverse roman chair – isometric

☐ Squats with ball against wall – isometric

☐ Bridge marching

☐ Upward dog

☐ Ball-Wall hip stability isometric

RETRAIN ACTIVITIES

RETRAIN Activity #1: _____

Better? _____   Worse? _____   Same? _____

Other: _____

Notes: _____

_____

RETRAIN Activity #2: _____

Better? _____   Worse? _____   Same? _____

Other: _____

Notes: _____

_____

RETRAIN Activity #3: _____

Better? _____   Worse? _____   Same? _____

Other: _____

Notes: _____

_____

PAIN LOCATION:

Use this figure to color or shade-in the area of your pain however you like.

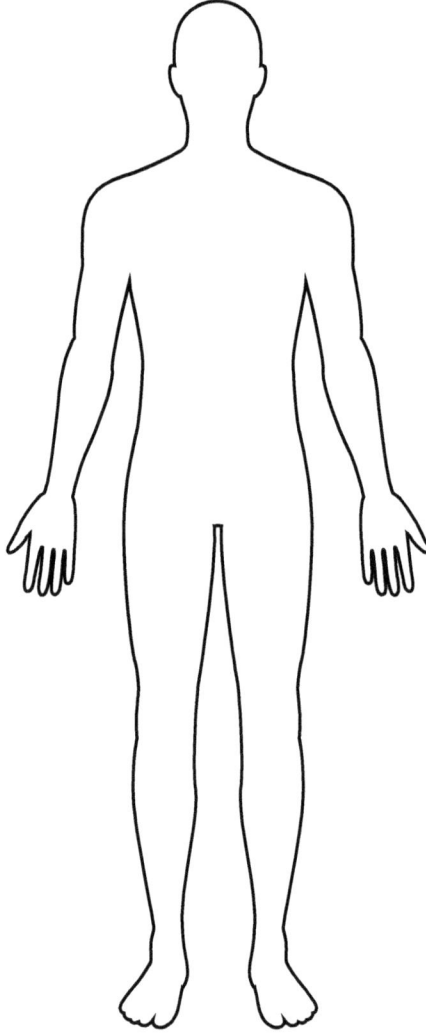

Quick Guide: Pain Locations

As seen in *The Everyday Pain Guide—Fix the Fire Damage*

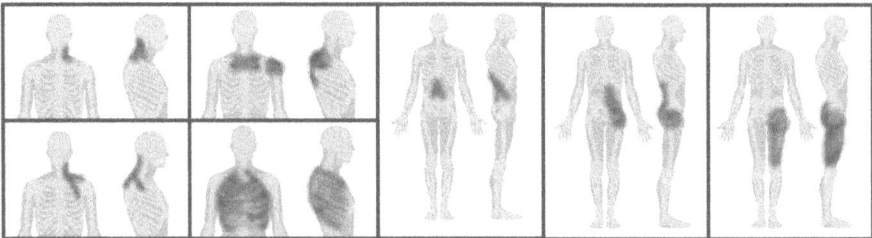

HOW MUCH PAIN TODAY?

Circle the face that best expresses your discomfort:

Wong-Baker FACES® Pain Rating Scale

0	2	4	6	8	10
No Pain	A Little Pain	A Little More Pain	Even More Pain	A Whole Lot Of Pain	Worst Pain

Notes:

_____

_____

_____

_____

_____

_____

_____

Remember to check out the Retrain phases of body chemistry and stress biology action plans.

RETRAIN – DAY 2

TODAY'S DATE: _____

Pick up to three of the following RETRAIN activities:

(Go to the Exercise Index in the Resources section at the back of the book, *Fix the Fire Damage*, to help you find these activities.)

☐ Posterior isometrics – neutral

☐ Posterior isometrics – at 45 deg.

☐ Shoulder shrug isometric

☐ Eagle arms pose

☐ Reach for the ceiling

☐ Wall plank

☐ Arm reach isometric

☐ External shoulder rotation isometric

☐ Triceps extension pulldown isometric

☐ Modified sphinx pose

☐ Shoulder shrug isometric – mid

☐ Bent over fly isometric – torso supported

☐ Inner thigh isometrics

☐ Superman isometrics with lower back and hip focus

☐ Clamshell isometric

☐ Hamstring stretch – active

☐ Reverse roman chair – isometric

☐ Squats with ball against wall – isometric

☐ Bridge marching

☐ Upward dog

☐ Ball-Wall hip stability isometric

RETRAIN ACTIVITIES

RETRAIN Activity #1: _____

Better? _____   Worse? _____   Same? _____

Other: _____

Notes: _____

_____

RETRAIN Activity #2: _____

Better? _____   Worse? _____   Same? _____

Other: _____

Notes: _____

_____

RETRAIN Activity #3: _____

Better? _____   Worse? _____   Same? _____

Other: _____

Notes: _____

_____

PAIN LOCATION:

Use this figure to color or shade-in the area of your pain however you like.

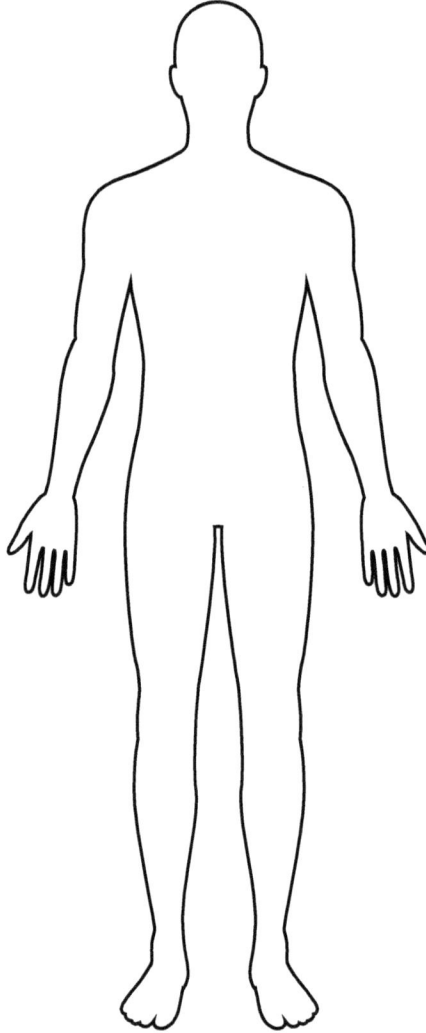

Quick Guide: Pain Locations

As seen in *The Everyday Pain Guide—Fix the Fire Damage*

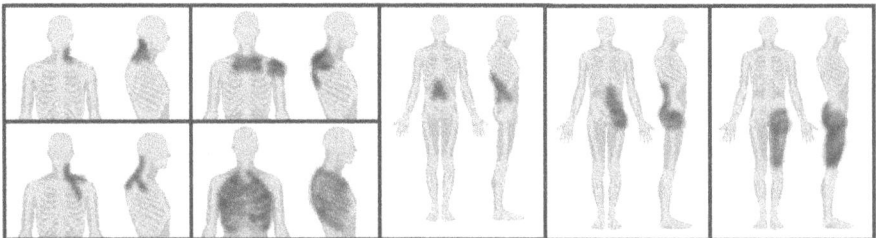

HOW MUCH PAIN TODAY?

Circle the face that best expresses your discomfort:

Wong-Baker FACES® Pain Rating Scale

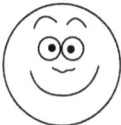 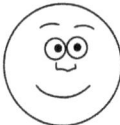 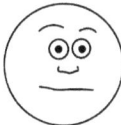 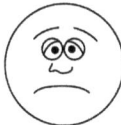 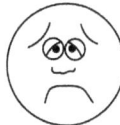 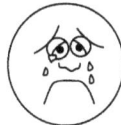

0	2	4	6	8	10
No Pain	A Little Pain	A Little More Pain	Even More Pain	A Whole Lot Of Pain	Worst Pain

Notes:

_____

_____

_____

_____

_____

_____

_____

Remember to check out the Retrain phases of body chemistry and stress biology action plans.

RETRAIN – DAY 3

TODAY'S DATE: _____

Pick up to three of the following RETRAIN activities:

(Go to the Exercise Index in the Resources section at the back of the book, *Fix the Fire Damage*, to help you find these activities.)

☐ Posterior isometrics – neutral

☐ Posterior isometrics – at 45 deg.

☐ Shoulder shrug isometric

☐ Eagle arms pose

☐ Reach for the ceiling

☐ Wall plank

☐ Arm reach isometric

☐ External shoulder rotation isometric

☐ Triceps extension pulldown isometric

☐ Modified sphinx pose

☐ Shoulder shrug isometric – mid

☐ Bent over fly isometric – torso supported

☐ Inner thigh isometrics

☐ Superman isometrics with lower back and hip focus

☐ Clamshell isometric

☐ Hamstring stretch – active

☐ Reverse roman chair – isometric

☐ Squats with ball against wall – isometric

☐ Bridge marching

☐ Upward dog

☐ Ball-Wall hip stability isometric

RETRAIN ACTIVITIES

RETRAIN Activity #1: _____

Better? _____   Worse? _____   Same? _____

Other: _____

Notes: _____

_____

RETRAIN Activity #2: _____

Better? _____   Worse? _____   Same? _____

Other: _____

Notes: _____

_____

RETRAIN Activity #3: _____

Better? _____   Worse? _____   Same? _____

Other: _____

Notes: _____

_____

PAIN LOCATION:

Use this figure to color or shade-in the area of your pain however you like.

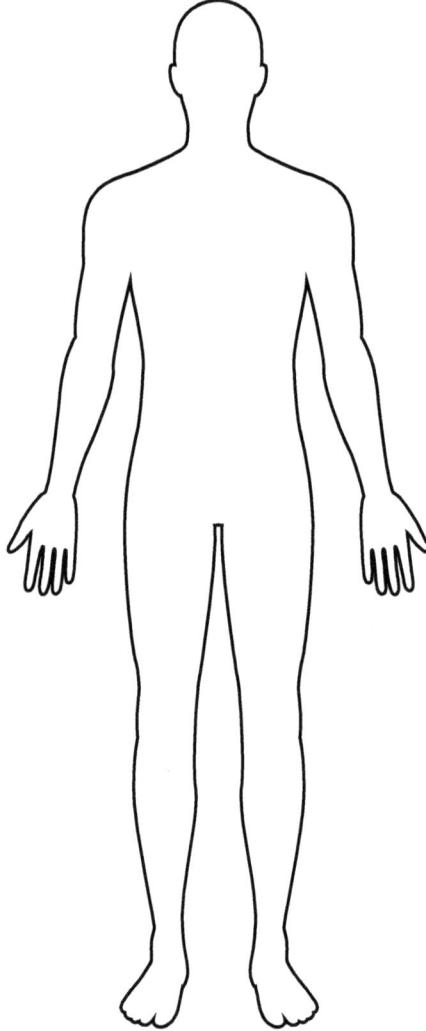

Quick Guide: Pain Locations

As seen in *The Everyday Pain Guide—Fix the Fire Damage*

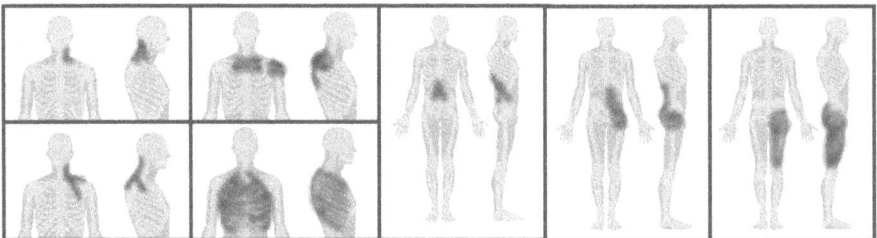

HOW MUCH PAIN TODAY?

Circle the face that best expresses your discomfort:

Wong-Baker FACES® Pain Rating Scale

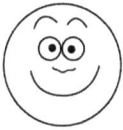 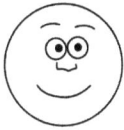 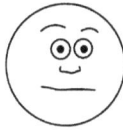 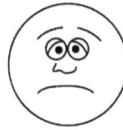 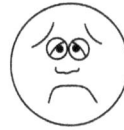 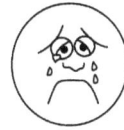

0	2	4	6	8	10
No Pain	A Little Pain	A Little More Pain	Even More Pain	A Whole Lot Of Pain	Worst Pain

Notes:

_____

_____

_____

_____

_____

_____

_____

Remember to check out the Retrain phases of body chemistry and stress biology action plans.

RETRAIN – DAY 4

TODAY'S DATE: _____

Pick up to three of the following RETRAIN activities:

(Go to the Exercise Index in the Resources section at the back of the book, Fix the Fire Damage, to help you find these activities.)

- [ ] Posterior isometrics – neutral
- [ ] Posterior isometrics – at 45 deg.
- [ ] Shoulder shrug isometric
- [ ] Eagle arms pose
- [ ] Reach for the ceiling
- [ ] Wall plank
- [ ] Arm reach isometric
- [ ] External shoulder rotation isometric
- [ ] Triceps extension pulldown isometric
- [ ] Modified sphinx pose
- [ ] Shoulder shrug isometric – mid

- [ ] Bent over fly isometric – torso supported
- [ ] Inner thigh isometrics
- [ ] Superman isometrics with lower back and hip focus
- [ ] Clamshell isometric
- [ ] Hamstring stretch – active
- [ ] Reverse roman chair – isometric
- [ ] Squats with ball against wall – isometric
- [ ] Bridge marching
- [ ] Upward dog
- [ ] Ball-Wall hip stability isometric

RETRAIN ACTIVITIES

RETRAIN Activity #1: _____

Better? _____   Worse? _____   Same? _____

Other: _____

Notes: _____

_____

RETRAIN Activity #2: _____

Better? _____   Worse? _____   Same? _____

Other: _____

Notes: _____

_____

RETRAIN Activity #3: _____

Better? _____   Worse? _____   Same? _____

Other: _____

Notes: _____

_____

PAIN LOCATION:

Use this figure to color or shade-in the area of your pain however you like.

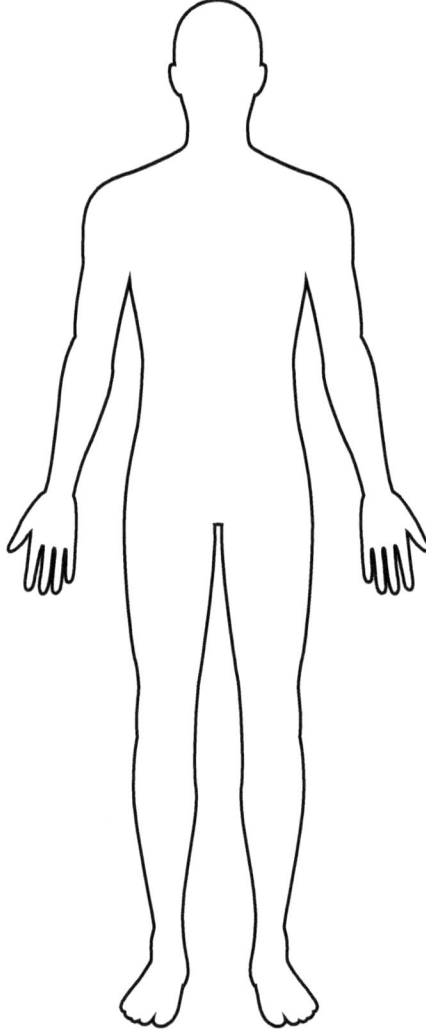

Quick Guide: Pain Locations

As seen in *The Everyday Pain Guide—Fix the Fire Damage*

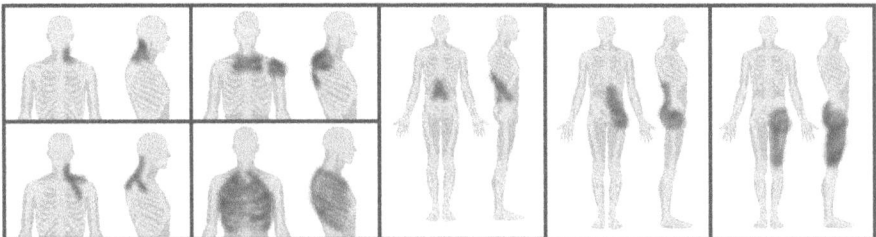

HOW MUCH PAIN TODAY?

Circle the face that best expresses your discomfort:

Wong-Baker FACES® Pain Rating Scale

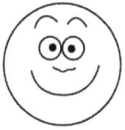 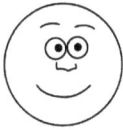 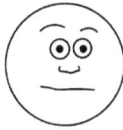 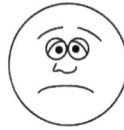 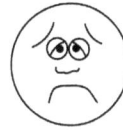 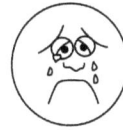

0	2	4	6	8	10
No Pain	A Little Pain	A Little More Pain	Even More Pain	A Whole Lot Of Pain	Worst Pain

Notes:

_____

_____

_____

_____

_____

_____

_____

_____

Remember to check out the Retrain phases of body chemistry and stress biology action plans.

RETRAIN – DAY 5

TODAY'S DATE: _____

Pick up to three of the following RETRAIN activities:

(Go to the Exercise Index in the Resources section at the back of the book, *Fix the Fire Damage*, to help you find these activities.)

- ☐ Posterior isometrics – neutral
- ☐ Posterior isometrics – at 45 deg.
- ☐ Shoulder shrug isometric
- ☐ Eagle arms pose
- ☐ Reach for the ceiling
- ☐ Wall plank
- ☐ Arm reach isometric
- ☐ External shoulder rotation isometric
- ☐ Triceps extension pulldown isometric
- ☐ Modified sphinx pose
- ☐ Shoulder shrug isometric – mid

- ☐ Bent over fly isometric – torso supported
- ☐ Inner thigh isometrics
- ☐ Superman isometrics with lower back and hip focus
- ☐ Clamshell isometric
- ☐ Hamstring stretch – active
- ☐ Reverse roman chair – isometric
- ☐ Squats with ball against wall – isometric
- ☐ Bridge marching
- ☐ Upward dog
- ☐ Ball-Wall hip stability isometric

RETRAIN ACTIVITIES

RETRAIN Activity #1: _____

Better? _____   Worse? _____   Same? _____

Other: _____

Notes: _____

_____

RETRAIN Activity #2: _____

Better? _____   Worse? _____   Same? _____

Other: _____

Notes: _____

_____

RETRAIN Activity #3: _____

Better? _____   Worse? _____   Same? _____

Other: _____

Notes: _____

_____

PAIN LOCATION:

Use this figure to color or shade-in the area of your pain however you like.

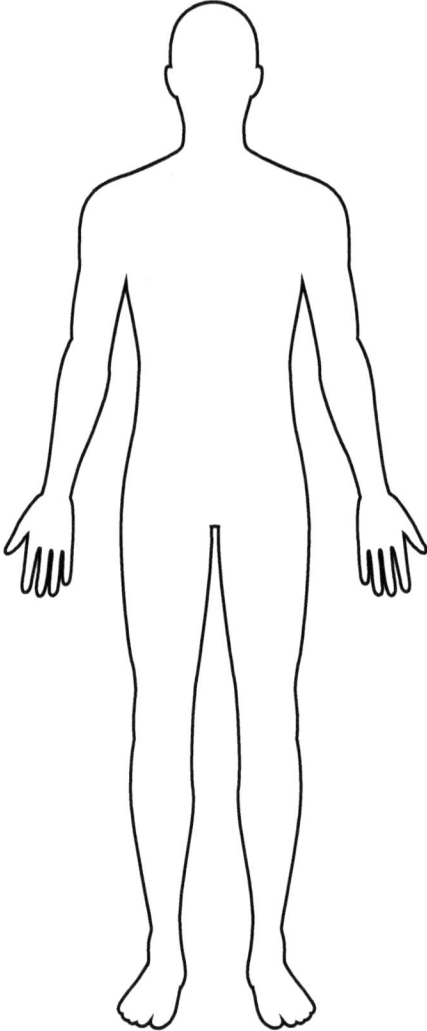

Quick Guide: Pain Locations

As seen in *The Everyday Pain Guide—Fix the Fire Damage*

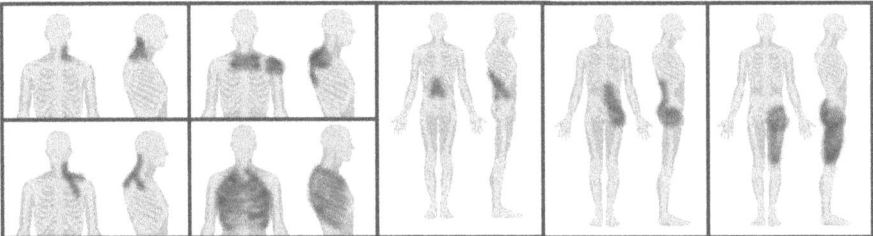

HOW MUCH PAIN TODAY?

Circle the face that best expresses your discomfort:

Wong-Baker FACES® Pain Rating Scale

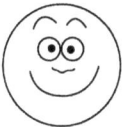 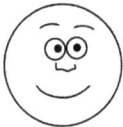 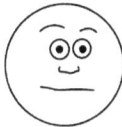 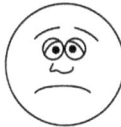 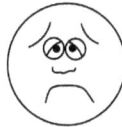 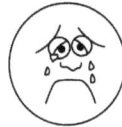

0	2	4	6	8	10
No Pain	A Little Pain	A Little More Pain	Even More Pain	A Whole Lot Of Pain	Worst Pain

Notes:

_____

_____

_____

_____

_____

_____

_____

Remember to check out the Retrain phases of body chemistry and stress biology action plans.

RETRAIN - DAY 6

TODAY'S DATE: _____

Pick up to three of the following RETRAIN activities:

(Go to the Exercise Index in the Resources section at the back of the book, *Fix the Fire Damage*, to help you find these activities.)

☐ Posterior isometrics – neutral

☐ Posterior isometrics – at 45 deg.

☐ Shoulder shrug isometric

☐ Eagle arms pose

☐ Reach for the ceiling

☐ Wall plank

☐ Arm reach isometric

☐ External shoulder rotation isometric

☐ Triceps extension pulldown isometric

☐ Modified sphinx pose

☐ Shoulder shrug isometric – mid

☐ Bent over fly isometric – torso supported

☐ Inner thigh isometrics

☐ Superman isometrics with lower back and hip focus

☐ Clamshell isometric

☐ Hamstring stretch – active

☐ Reverse roman chair – isometric

☐ Squats with ball against wall – isometric

☐ Bridge marching

☐ Upward dog

☐ Ball-Wall hip stability isometric

RETRAIN ACTIVITIES

RETRAIN Activity #1: _____

Better? _____ Worse? _____ Same? _____

Other: _____

Notes: _____

_____

RETRAIN Activity #2: _____

Better? _____ Worse? _____ Same? _____

Other: _____

Notes: _____

_____

RETRAIN Activity #3: _____

Better? _____ Worse? _____ Same? _____

Other: _____

Notes: _____

_____

PAIN LOCATION:
Use this figure to color or shade-in the area of your pain however you like.

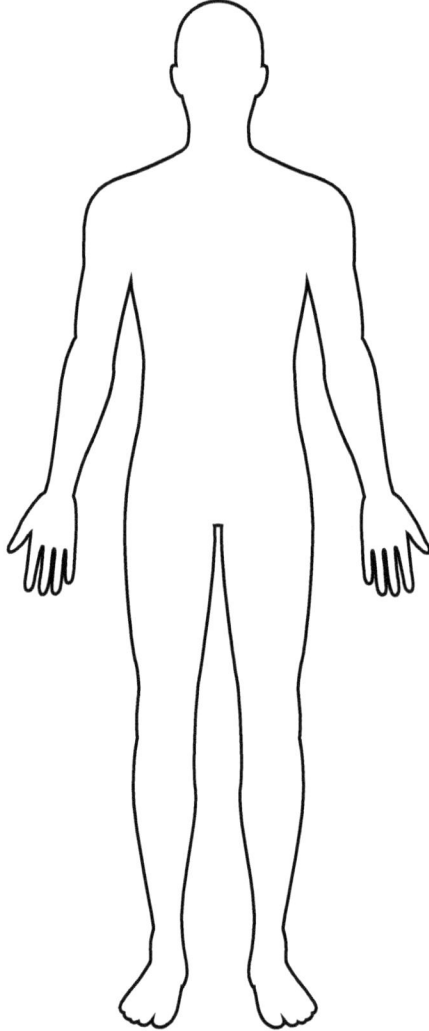

Quick Guide: Pain Locations
As seen in *The Everyday Pain Guide—Fix the Fire Damage*

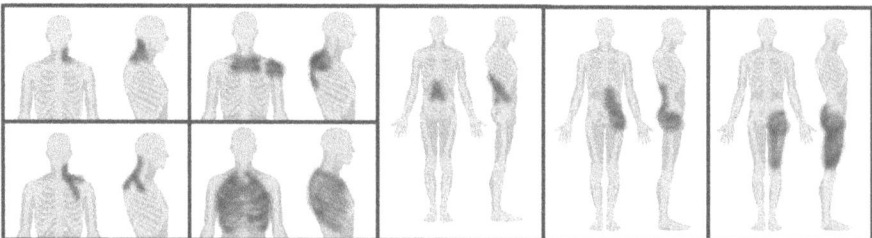

HOW MUCH PAIN TODAY?

Circle the face that best expresses your discomfort:

Wong-Baker FACES® Pain Rating Scale

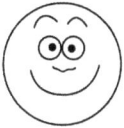 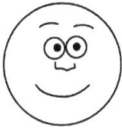 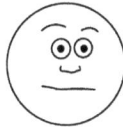 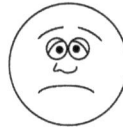 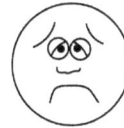 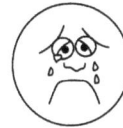

0	2	4	6	8	10
No Pain	A Little Pain	A Little More Pain	Even More Pain	A Whole Lot Of Pain	Worst Pain

Notes:

_____

_____

_____

_____

_____

_____

_____

Remember to check out the Retrain phases of body chemistry and stress biology action plans.

RETRAIN – DAY 7

TODAY'S DATE: _____

Pick up to three of the following RETRAIN activities:

(Go to the Exercise Index in the Resources section at the back of the book, *Fix the Fire Damage*, to help you find these activities.)

- ☐ Posterior isometrics – neutral
- ☐ Posterior isometrics – at 45 deg.
- ☐ Shoulder shrug isometric
- ☐ Eagle arms pose
- ☐ Reach for the ceiling
- ☐ Wall plank
- ☐ Arm reach isometric
- ☐ External shoulder rotation isometric
- ☐ Triceps extension pulldown isometric
- ☐ Modified sphinx pose
- ☐ Shoulder shrug isometric – mid

- ☐ Bent over fly isometric – torso supported
- ☐ Inner thigh isometrics
- ☐ Superman isometrics with lower back and hip focus
- ☐ Clamshell isometric
- ☐ Hamstring stretch – active
- ☐ Reverse roman chair – isometric
- ☐ Squats with ball against wall – isometric
- ☐ Bridge marching
- ☐ Upward dog
- ☐ Ball-Wall hip stability isometric

RETRAIN ACTIVITIES

RETRAIN Activity #1: _____

Better? _____   Worse? _____   Same? _____

Other: _____

Notes: _____

_____

RETRAIN Activity #2: _____

Better? _____   Worse? _____   Same? _____

Other: _____

Notes: _____

_____

RETRAIN Activity #3: _____

Better? _____   Worse? _____   Same? _____

Other: _____

Notes: _____

_____

PAIN LOCATION:

Use this figure to color or shade-in the area of your pain however you like.

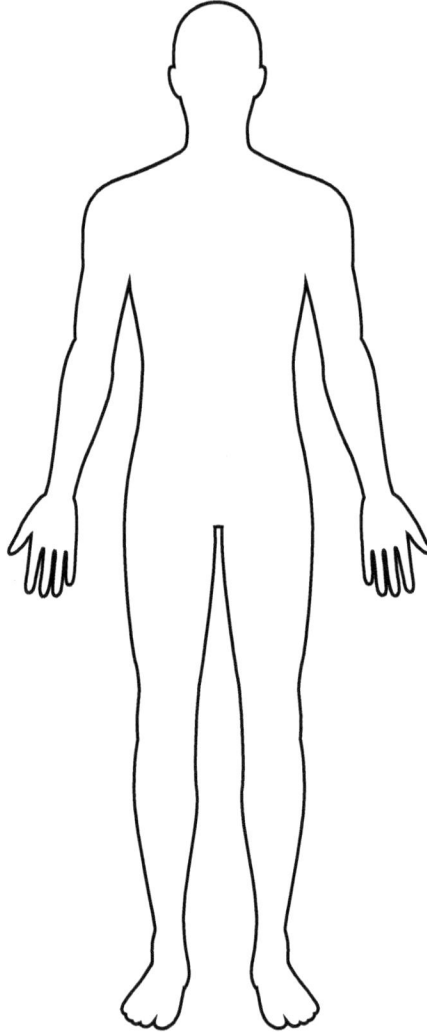

Quick Guide: Pain Locations

As seen in *The Everyday Pain Guide—Fix the Fire Damage*

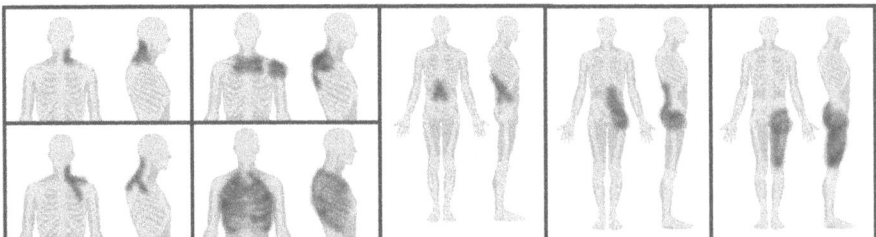

HOW MUCH PAIN TODAY?

Circle the face that best expresses your discomfort:

Wong-Baker FACES® Pain Rating Scale

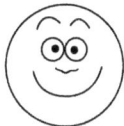 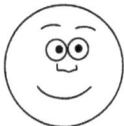 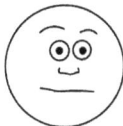 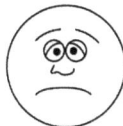 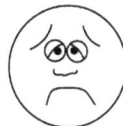 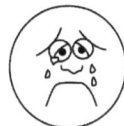

0	2	4	6	8	10
No Pain	A Little Pain	A Little More Pain	Even More Pain	A Whole Lot Of Pain	Worst Pain

Notes:

_____

_____

_____

_____

_____

_____

_____

Remember to check out the Retrain phases of body chemistry and stress biology action plans.

Have you completed the Retrain phase of action?

Q: Do you still feel the pain here and there, but you're able to complete your daily tasks uninterrupted without special modifications?

Circle one: Yes / No

Details:_____

_____

_____

_____

_____

_____

_____

_____

_____

_____

_____

Q: Do you still feel some pain in bed at night, but no longer have to think too much about your positioning and pillow support to fall asleep?

Circle one: Yes / No

Details:_____

_____

_____

_____

_____

_____

_____

_____

If you answered YES to any of the questions, then you may need to continue with your Retrain activities even if you are ready to move forward. Take it slow.

Are you ready for the next phase of action - Reinforce?

Q: Are you itching to get back to your usual activities?

Circle one: Yes / No

Details:_____

_____

_____

_____

_____

Q: Are you getting bored or restless with the Release and Retrain activities?

Circle one: Yes / No

Details:_____

_____

_____

_____

_____

Q: Have you had 5-7 consecutive days of no pain reminders at all?

Circle one: Yes / No

Details:_____

_____

_____

_____

_____

_____

If you answered YES to all of the questions, then you are ready to try the Reinforce activities.

Consider revisiting the Release phase activities - it's natural to have days when it feels like you've taken a step or two backwards.

Stay open to peeling back to the Retrain (isometric) versions of the Reinforce activities.

"Success is not final,

failure is not fatal:

it is the courage

to continue that

counts."

—Winston Churchill

My *Reinforce* Action Steps

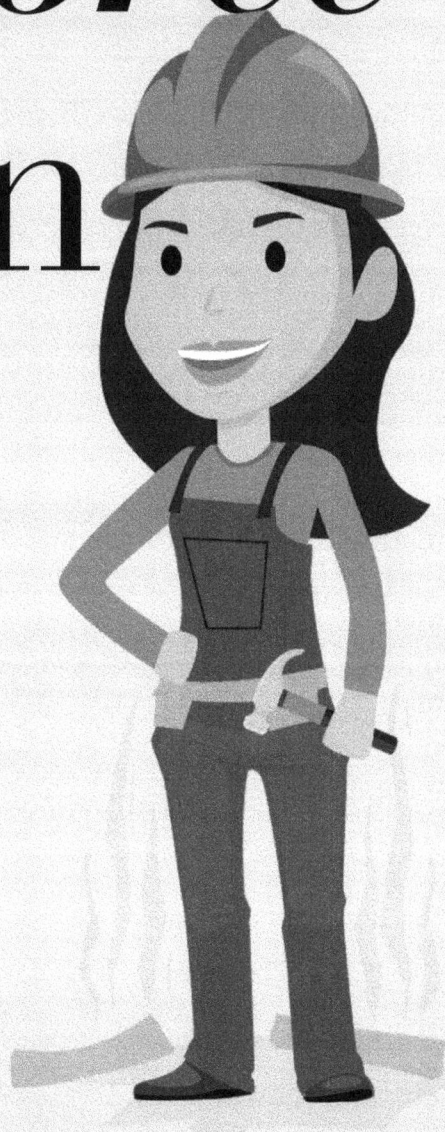

THE CHECK IN

How are you feeling?

TODAY'S DATE: _____

PAIN LOCATION:
(circle one)

Neck   Neck/Shoulder   Shoulder/Upper Back   Mid Back/Torso/Ribs

Low Back   Low Back/Hip   Hip/Buttock/Thigh

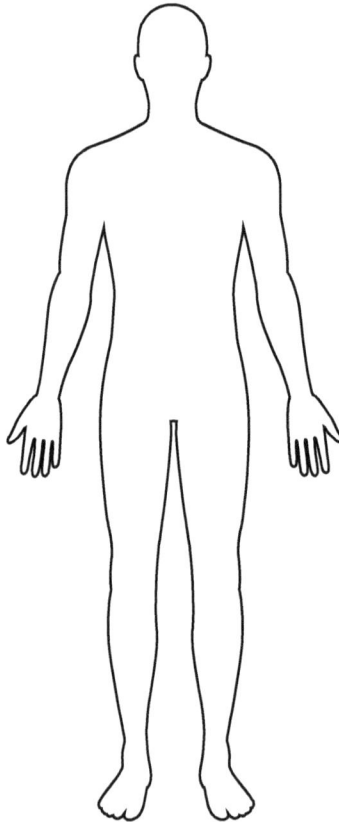

Use this figure to color or shade-in the area of your pain however you like.

HOW MUCH PAIN TODAY?

Circle the face below that best expresses your discomfort:

Wong-Baker FACES® Pain Rating Scale

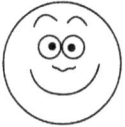 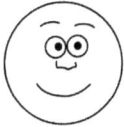 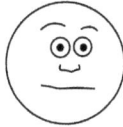 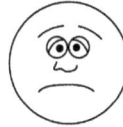 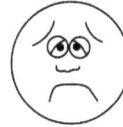 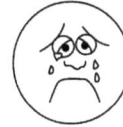

0	**2**	**4**	**6**	**8**	**10**
No Pain	A Little Pain	A Little More Pain	Even More Pain	A Whole Lot Of Pain	Worst Pain

- If you circled #4, consider continuing with your Retrain actions while proceeding.
- If you circled #6 or higher, please return to Release & Retrain for at least another week before proceeding.

Notes:

_____

_____

_____

_____

_____

_____

My pain feels:
(circle all that apply)

Sharp   Stabbing   Achy   Tingly   Throbbing

Grabbing   Tightness   Pinching

Other/More Details: _____

_____

_____

_____

When do I notice it the *most*?
(circle all that apply)

Sitting   Standing still   Walking   Getting up from sitting

Lying on my back   Lying on my belly   Lying on my RIGHT side

Lying on my LEFT side   Driving the car   Mornings

Before bed   Middle of the night

Other/More Details: _____

_____

_____

_____

When do I notice it *less*?
(circle all that apply)

Sitting   Standing still   Walking   Getting up from sitting

Lying on my back   Lying on my belly   Lying on my RIGHT side

Lying on my LEFT side   Driving the car   Mornings

Before bed   Middle of the night

Other/More Details: _____

_____

_____

_____

_____

Medication used:
(circle all that apply)

Ibuprofen (Motrin/Advil)   Naproxen (Aleve)   Acetaminophen (Tylenol)

Other/Prescription: _____

_____

How much? _____

_____

☐ Some Relief?   ☐ Total Relief?   ☐ No Relief?

REINFORCE!

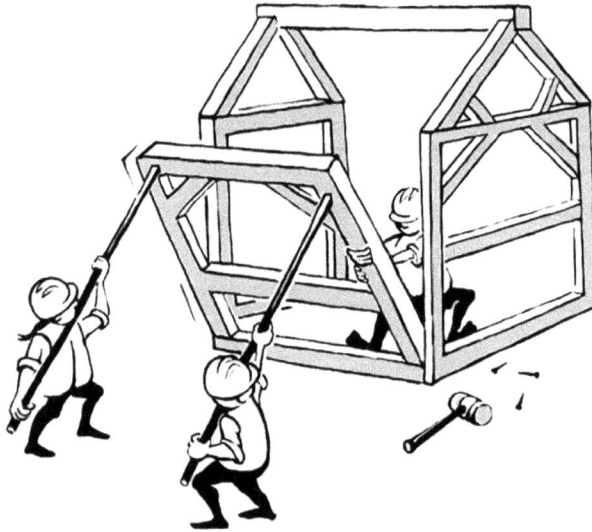

Build a strong foundation creating physical strength and stability while nurturing supportive habits of self-care.

Q: *What's* being reinforced?

A: **Coordination, strength, and stability for future resilience against flare-ups**

Q: *How* will coordination, strength, and stability be reinforced?

A: **By building on the strategic isometrics from Action Phase 2: Retrain**

NEXT STEPS:

1. Return to the action plan for your pain location in *The Everyday Pain Guide – Fix the Fire Damage.*

2. This time try all **Reinforce** activities associated with your pain location.

3. Pick up to three **Reinforce** activities for daily use and record your progress in the following pages…

Body Mechanics Reinforce techniques will help you nurture the now newly revived areas of your brain-body connection. You will begin to create strength specific to your need and the area of pain. Gently increasing strength in this targeted way will help you to prevent future flare-ups and to become inflammation fireproof. The goal of the Reinforce phase is to strengthen and prepare you for life's demands.

Reinforce action steps are important tactics for the final phases of repair as you move into the third stage of healing and prepare to become more independent from supportive treatments like acupuncture, chiropractic, or physical therapy. When you use Reinforce activities for this final phase, you're implementing strategies that are designed to keep the pain from coming back.

It's essential to implement Reinforce action steps while pain and inflammation are still fresh in your memory, even if no longer in your body. The occasional hints or reminders of recent pain act as important guides to help us refine our long-term plan for protection against reinjury.

Notes:

_____

_____

_____

_____

_____

_____

_____

_____

_____

_____

_____

_____

_____

_____

_____

_____

Reinforce
Activities

Week One

TODAY'S DATE: _____

Pick up to three of the following REINFORCE activities:

(Go to the Exercise Index in the Resources section at the back of the book, *Fix the Fire Damage*, to help you find these activities.)

☐ Plank hover (intermediate)

☐ Plank hover (advanced)

☐ Plank hover with inflate/deflate repetitions (advanced)

☐ Side plank (advanced)

☐ Downward dog with upward gaze (advanced)

☐ Neck turn and head nod

☐ Superman isometrics with neck focus

☐ Superman isometrics

☐ Tiny arm circles

☐ External shoulder rotation – repetitions + resistance (lying down)

☐ External shoulder rotation – repetitions + resistance (standing)

☐ Triceps extension pulldowns – repetitions + resistance

☐ Reach for the ceiling – repetitions + resistance

☐ Arm shoulder circles (forward rotation)

☐ Bent over fly

☐ Bench press with extra push

☐ Monster walk

☐ Clamshell pulse

☐ Reverse roman chair repetitions

☐ Dead bug – beginner

☐ Dead bug – intermediate

☐ Forearm plank – marching

☐ Bird dog

☐ Squat with side kick

☐ Ball-wall hip stability

☐ Supine hip circles – knee bent

☐ Supine hip circles – straight leg

REINFORCE ACTIVITIES

REINFORCE Activity #1: _____

Better? _____   Worse? _____   Same? _____

Other: _____

Notes: _____

_____

REINFORCE Activity #2: _____

Better? _____   Worse? _____   Same? _____

Other: _____

Notes: _____

_____

REINFORCE Activity #3: _____

Better? _____   Worse? _____   Same? _____

Other: _____

Notes: _____

_____

PAIN LOCATION:

Use this figure to color or shade-in the area of your pain however you like.

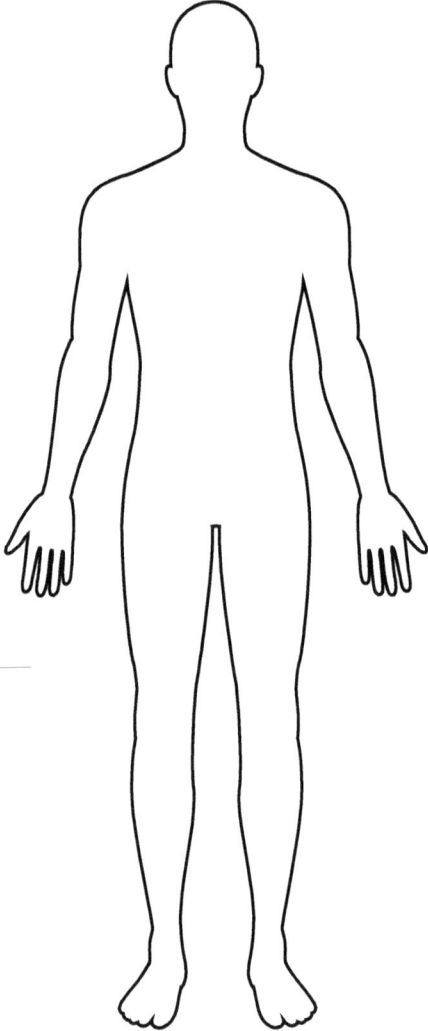

Quick Guide: Pain Locations

As seen in *The Everyday Pain Guide—Fix the Fire Damage*

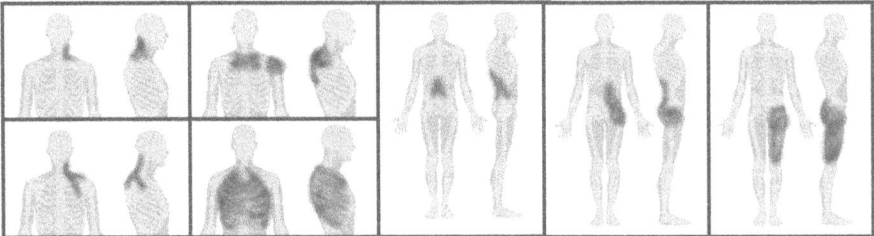

HOW MUCH PAIN TODAY?

Circle the face that best expresses your discomfort:

Wong-Baker FACES® Pain Rating Scale

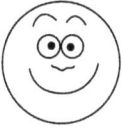 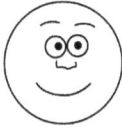 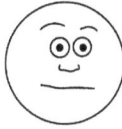 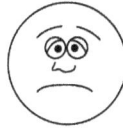 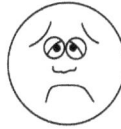 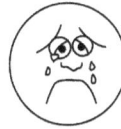

0	**2**	**4**	**6**	**8**	**10**
No Pain	A Little Pain	A Little More Pain	Even More Pain	A Whole Lot Of Pain	Worst Pain

Notes:

_____

_____

_____

_____

_____

_____

_____

Remember to check out the Reinforce phases of body chemistry and stress biology action plans.

REINFORCE – DAY 2

TODAY'S DATE: _____

Pick up to three of the following REINFORCE activities:

(Go to the Exercise Index in the Resources section at the back of the book, *Fix the Fire Damage*, to help you find these activities.)

- ☐ Plank hover (intermediate)
- ☐ Plank hover (advanced)
- ☐ Plank hover with inflate/deflate repetitions (advanced)
- ☐ Side plank (advanced)
- ☐ Downward dog with upward gaze (advanced)
- ☐ Neck turn and head nod
- ☐ Superman isometrics with neck focus
- ☐ Superman isometrics
- ☐ Tiny arm circles
- ☐ External shoulder rotation – repetitions + resistance (lying down)
- ☐ External shoulder rotation – repetitions + resistance (standing)
- ☐ Triceps extension pulldowns – repetitions + resistance
- ☐ Reach for the ceiling – repetitions + resistance
- ☐ Arm shoulder circles (forward rotation)

- ☐ Bent over fly
- ☐ Bench press with extra push
- ☐ Monster walk
- ☐ Clamshell pulse
- ☐ Reverse roman chair repetitions
- ☐ Dead bug – beginner
- ☐ Dead bug – intermediate
- ☐ Forearm plank – marching
- ☐ Bird dog
- ☐ Squat with side kick
- ☐ Ball-wall hip stability
- ☐ Supine hip circles – knee bent
- ☐ Supine hip circles – straight leg

REINFORCE ACTIVITIES

REINFORCE Activity #1: _____

Better? _____   Worse? _____   Same? _____

Other: _____

Notes: _____

_____

REINFORCE Activity #2: _____

Better? _____   Worse? _____   Same? _____

Other: _____

Notes: _____

_____

REINFORCE Activity #3: _____

Better? _____   Worse? _____   Same? _____

Other: _____

Notes: _____

_____

PAIN LOCATION:

Use this figure to color or shade-in the area of your pain however you like.

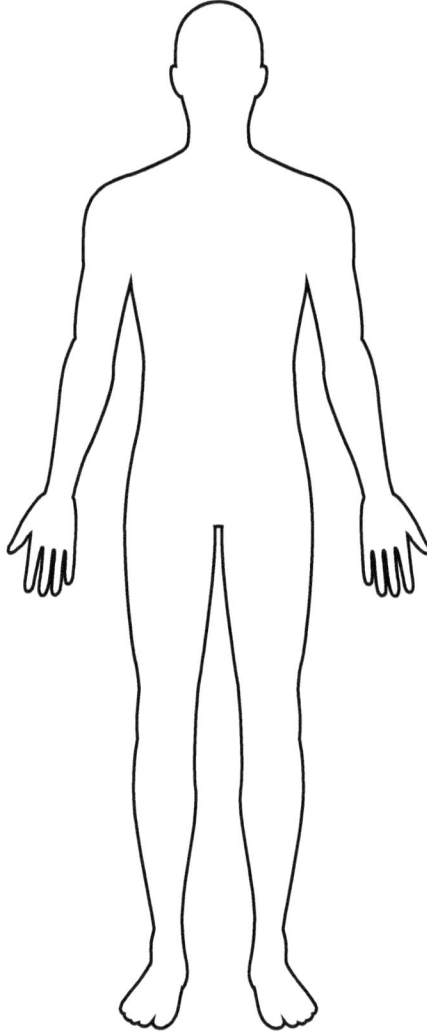

Quick Guide: Pain Locations

As seen in *The Everyday Pain Guide—Fix the Fire Damage*

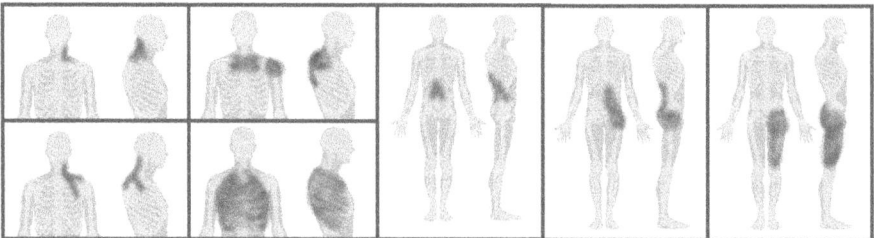

HOW MUCH PAIN TODAY?

Circle the face that best expresses your discomfort:

Wong-Baker FACES® Pain Rating Scale

0	2	4	6	8	10
No Pain	A Little Pain	A Little More Pain	Even More Pain	A Whole Lot Of Pain	Worst Pain

Notes:

_____

_____

_____

_____

_____

_____

_____

Remember to check out the Reinforce phases of body chemistry and stress biology action plans.

TODAY'S DATE: _____

Pick up to three of the following REINFORCE activities:

(Go to the Exercise Index in the Resources section at the back of the book, *Fix the Fire Damage*, to help you find these activities.)

☐ Plank hover (intermediate)

☐ Plank hover (advanced)

☐ Plank hover with inflate/deflate repetitions (advanced)

☐ Side plank (advanced)

☐ Downward dog with upward gaze (advanced)

☐ Neck turn and head nod

☐ Superman isometrics with neck focus

☐ Superman isometrics

☐ Tiny arm circles

☐ External shoulder rotation – repetitions + resistance (lying down)

☐ External shoulder rotation – repetitions + resistance (standing)

☐ Triceps extension pulldowns – repetitions + resistance

☐ Reach for the ceiling – repetitions + resistance

☐ Arm shoulder circles (forward rotation)

☐ Bent over fly

☐ Bench press with extra push

☐ Monster walk

☐ Clamshell pulse

☐ Reverse roman chair repetitions

☐ Dead bug – beginner

☐ Dead bug – intermediate

☐ Forearm plank – marching

☐ Bird dog

☐ Squat with side kick

☐ Ball-wall hip stability

☐ Supine hip circles – knee bent

☐ Supine hip circles – straight leg

REINFORCE ACTIVITIES

REINFORCE Activity #1: _____

Better? _____   Worse? _____   Same? _____

Other: _____

Notes: _____

_____

REINFORCE Activity #2: _____

Better? _____   Worse? _____   Same? _____

Other: _____

Notes: _____

_____

REINFORCE Activity #3: _____

Better? _____   Worse? _____   Same? _____

Other: _____

Notes: _____

_____

PAIN LOCATION:

Use this figure to color or shade-in the area of your pain however you like.

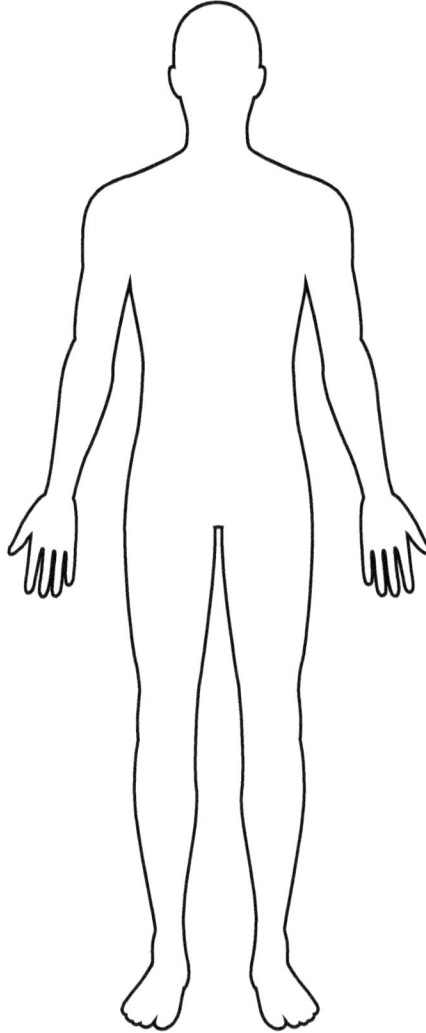

Quick Guide: Pain Locations

As seen in *The Everyday Pain Guide—Fix the Fire Damage*

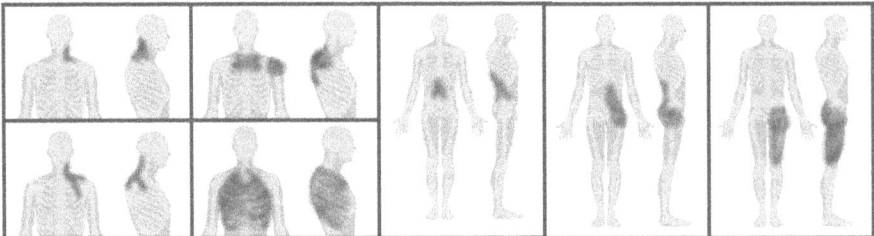

HOW MUCH PAIN TODAY?

Circle the face that best expresses your discomfort:

Wong-Baker FACES® Pain Rating Scale

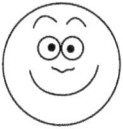 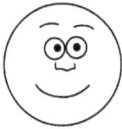 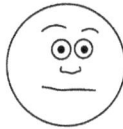 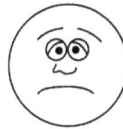 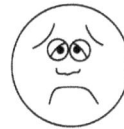 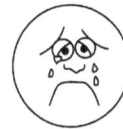

0	**2**	**4**	**6**	**8**	**10**
No Pain	A Little Pain	A Little More Pain	Even More Pain	A Whole Lot Of Pain	Worst Pain

Notes:

_____

_____

_____

_____

_____

_____

_____

Remember to check out the Reinforce phases of body chemistry and stress biology action plans.

REINFORCE – DAY 4

TODAY'S DATE: _____

Pick up to three of the following REINFORCE activities:

(Go to the Exercise Index in the Resources section at the back of the book, *Fix the Fire Damage*, to help you find these activities.)

- ☐ Plank hover (intermediate)
- ☐ Plank hover (advanced)
- ☐ Plank hover with inflate/deflate repetitions (advanced)
- ☐ Side plank (advanced)
- ☐ Downward dog with upward gaze (advanced)
- ☐ Neck turn and head nod
- ☐ Superman isometrics with neck focus
- ☐ Superman isometrics
- ☐ Tiny arm circles
- ☐ External shoulder rotation – repetitions + resistance (lying down)
- ☐ External shoulder rotation – repetitions + resistance (standing)
- ☐ Triceps extension pulldowns – repetitions + resistance
- ☐ Reach for the ceiling – repetitions + resistance
- ☐ Arm shoulder circles (forward rotation)

- ☐ Bent over fly
- ☐ Bench press with extra push
- ☐ Monster walk
- ☐ Clamshell pulse
- ☐ Reverse roman chair repetitions
- ☐ Dead bug – beginner
- ☐ Dead bug – intermediate
- ☐ Forearm plank – marching
- ☐ Bird dog
- ☐ Squat with side kick
- ☐ Ball-wall hip stability
- ☐ Supine hip circles – knee bent
- ☐ Supine hip circles – straight leg

REINFORCE ACTIVITIES

REINFORCE Activity #1: _____

Better? _____   Worse? _____   Same? _____

Other: _____

Notes: _____

_____

REINFORCE Activity #2: _____

Better? _____   Worse? _____   Same? _____

Other: _____

Notes: _____

_____

REINFORCE Activity #3: _____

Better? _____   Worse? _____   Same? _____

Other: _____

Notes: _____

_____

PAIN LOCATION:

Use this figure to color or shade-in the area of your pain however you like.

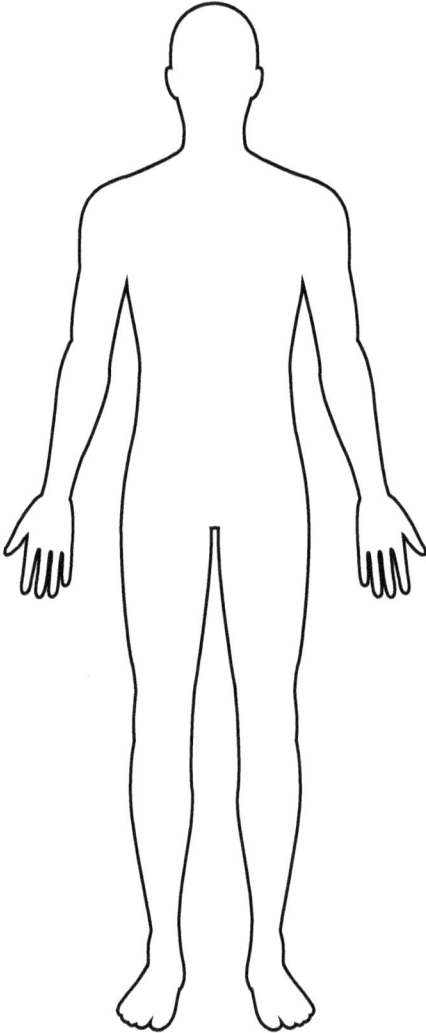

Quick Guide: Pain Locations

As seen in *The Everyday Pain Guide—Fix the Fire Damage*

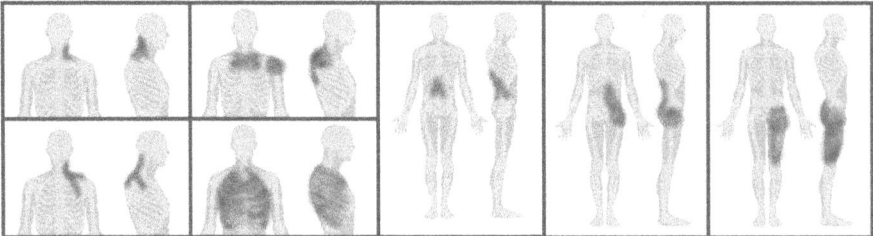

HOW MUCH PAIN TODAY?

Circle the face that best expresses your discomfort:

Wong-Baker FACES® Pain Rating Scale

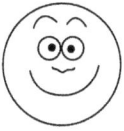 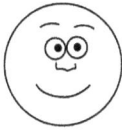 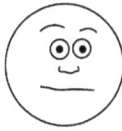 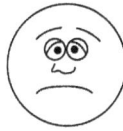 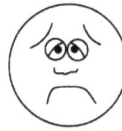 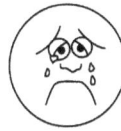

0	2	4	6	8	10
No Pain	A Little Pain	A Little More Pain	Even More Pain	A Whole Lot Of Pain	Worst Pain

Notes:

_____

_____

_____

_____

_____

_____

_____

_____

Remember to check out the Reinforce phases of body chemistry and stress biology action plans.

TODAY'S DATE: _____

Pick up to three of the following REINFORCE activities:

(Go to the Exercise Index in the Resources section at the back of the book, Fix the Fire Damage, to help you find these activities.)

- ☐ Plank hover (intermediate)
- ☐ Plank hover (advanced)
- ☐ Plank hover with inflate/deflate repetitions (advanced)
- ☐ Side plank (advanced)
- ☐ Downward dog with upward gaze (advanced)
- ☐ Neck turn and head nod
- ☐ Superman isometrics with neck focus
- ☐ Superman isometrics
- ☐ Tiny arm circles
- ☐ External shoulder rotation – repetitions + resistance (lying down)
- ☐ External shoulder rotation – repetitions + resistance (standing)
- ☐ Triceps extension pulldowns – repetitions + resistance
- ☐ Reach for the ceiling – repetitions + resistance
- ☐ Arm shoulder circles (forward rotation)

- ☐ Bent over fly
- ☐ Bench press with extra push
- ☐ Monster walk
- ☐ Clamshell pulse
- ☐ Reverse roman chair repetitions
- ☐ Dead bug – beginner
- ☐ Dead bug – intermediate
- ☐ Forearm plank – marching
- ☐ Bird dog
- ☐ Squat with side kick
- ☐ Ball-wall hip stability
- ☐ Supine hip circles – knee bent
- ☐ Supine hip circles – straight leg

REINFORCE ACTIVITIES

REINFORCE Activity #1: _____

Better? _____   Worse? _____   Same? _____

Other: _____

Notes: _____

_____

REINFORCE Activity #2: _____

Better? _____   Worse? _____   Same? _____

Other: _____

Notes: _____

_____

REINFORCE Activity #3: _____

Better? _____   Worse? _____   Same? _____

Other: _____

Notes: _____

_____

PAIN LOCATION:

Use this figure to color or shade-in the area of your pain however you like.

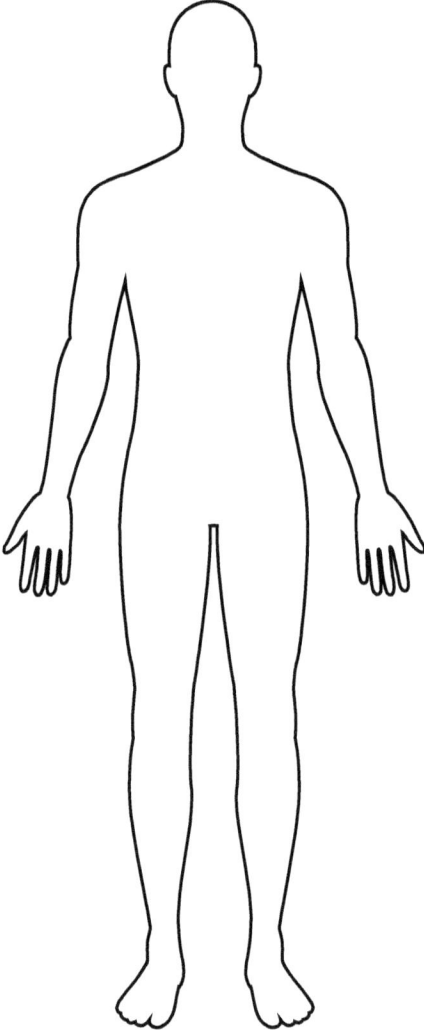

Quick Guide: Pain Locations

As seen in *The Everyday Pain Guide—Fix the Fire Damage*

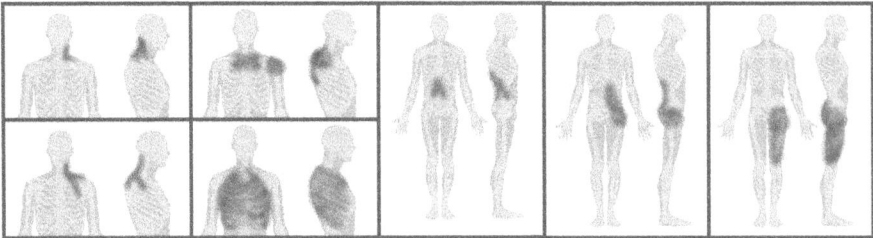

HOW MUCH PAIN TODAY?

Circle the face that best expresses your discomfort:

Wong-Baker FACES® Pain Rating Scale

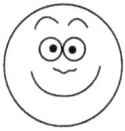 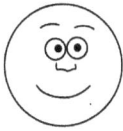 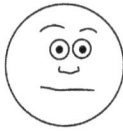 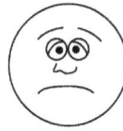 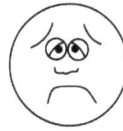 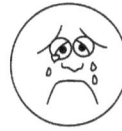

0	2	4	6	8	10
No Pain	A Little Pain	A Little More Pain	Even More Pain	A Whole Lot Of Pain	Worst Pain

Notes:

_____

_____

_____

_____

_____

_____

_____

Remember to check out the Reinforce phases of body chemistry and stress biology action plans.

REINFORCE – DAY 6

TODAY'S DATE: _____

Pick up to three of the following REINFORCE activities:

(Go to the Exercise Index in the Resources section at the back of the book, *Fix the Fire Damage*, to help you find these activities.)

- [ ] Plank hover (intermediate)
- [ ] Plank hover (advanced)
- [ ] Plank hover with inflate/deflate repetitions (advanced)
- [ ] Side plank (advanced)
- [ ] Downward dog with upward gaze (advanced)
- [ ] Neck turn and head nod
- [ ] Superman isometrics with neck focus
- [ ] Superman isometrics
- [ ] Tiny arm circles
- [ ] External shoulder rotation – repetitions + resistance (lying down)
- [ ] External shoulder rotation – repetitions + resistance (standing)
- [ ] Triceps extension pulldowns – repetitions + resistance
- [ ] Reach for the ceiling – repetitions + resistance
- [ ] Arm shoulder circles (forward rotation)

- [ ] Bent over fly
- [ ] Bench press with extra push
- [ ] Monster walk
- [ ] Clamshell pulse
- [ ] Reverse roman chair repetitions
- [ ] Dead bug – beginner
- [ ] Dead bug – intermediate
- [ ] Forearm plank – marching
- [ ] Bird dog
- [ ] Squat with side kick
- [ ] Ball-wall hip stability
- [ ] Supine hip circles – knee bent
- [ ] Supine hip circles – straight leg

REINFORCE ACTIVITIES

REINFORCE Activity #1: _____

Better? _____   Worse? _____   Same? _____

Other: _____

Notes: _____

_____

REINFORCE Activity #2: _____

Better? _____   Worse? _____   Same? _____

Other: _____

Notes: _____

_____

REINFORCE Activity #3: _____

Better? _____   Worse? _____   Same? _____

Other: _____

Notes: _____

_____

PAIN LOCATION:

Use this figure to color or shade-in the area of your pain however you like.

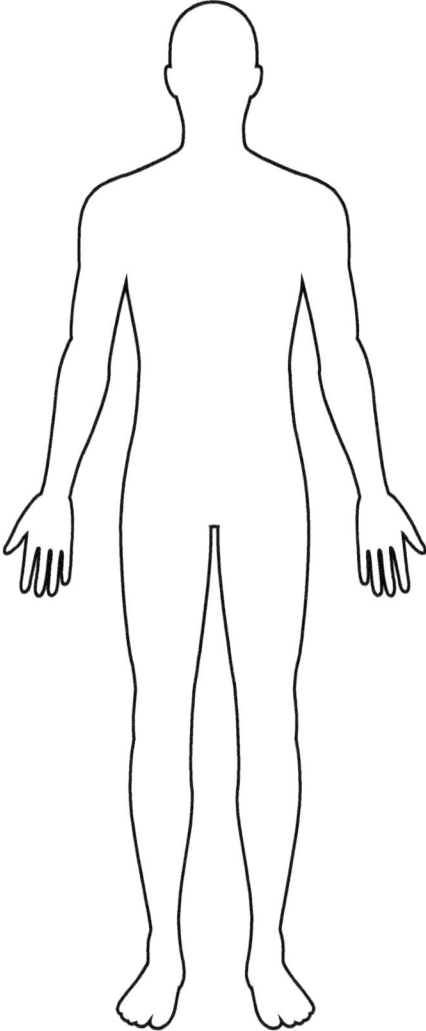

Quick Guide: Pain Locations

As seen in *The Everyday Pain Guide—Fix the Fire Damage*

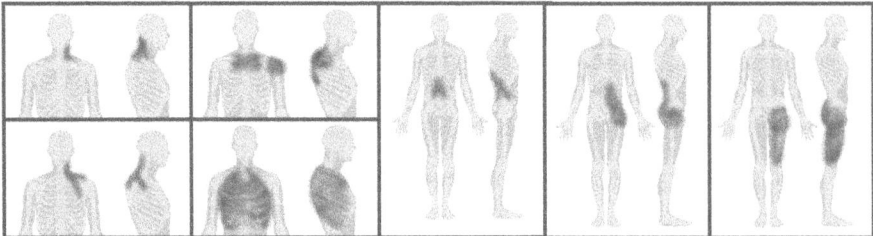

HOW MUCH PAIN TODAY?

Circle the face that best expresses your discomfort:

Wong-Baker FACES® Pain Rating Scale

0	2	4	6	8	10
No Pain	A Little Pain	A Little More Pain	Even More Pain	A Whole Lot Of Pain	Worst Pain

Notes:

_____

_____

_____

_____

_____

_____

_____

Remember to check out the Reinforce phases of body chemistry and stress biology action plans.

REINFORCE – DAY 7

TODAY'S DATE: _____

Pick up to three of the following REINFORCE activities:

(Go to the Exercise Index in the Resources section at the back of the book, *Fix the Fire Damage*, to help you find these activities.)

☐ Plank hover (intermediate)

☐ Plank hover (advanced)

☐ Plank hover with inflate/deflate repetitions (advanced)

☐ Side plank (advanced)

☐ Downward dog with upward gaze (advanced)

☐ Neck turn and head nod

☐ Superman isometrics with neck focus

☐ Superman isometrics

☐ Tiny arm circles

☐ External shoulder rotation – repetitions + resistance (lying down)

☐ External shoulder rotation – repetitions + resistance (standing)

☐ Triceps extension pulldowns – repetitions + resistance

☐ Reach for the ceiling – repetitions + resistance

☐ Arm shoulder circles (forward rotation)

☐ Bent over fly

☐ Bench press with extra push

☐ Monster walk

☐ Clamshell pulse

☐ Reverse roman chair repetitions

☐ Dead bug – beginner

☐ Dead bug – intermediate

☐ Forearm plank – marching

☐ Bird dog

☐ Squat with side kick

☐ Ball-wall hip stability

☐ Supine hip circles – knee bent

☐ Supine hip circles – straight leg

REINFORCE ACTIVITIES

REINFORCE Activity #1: _____

Better? _____   Worse? _____   Same? _____

Other: _____

Notes: _____

_____

REINFORCE Activity #2: _____

Better? _____   Worse? _____   Same? _____

Other: _____

Notes: _____

_____

REINFORCE Activity #3: _____

Better? _____   Worse? _____   Same? _____

Other: _____

Notes: _____

_____

PAIN LOCATION:

Use this figure to color or shade-in the area of your pain however you like.

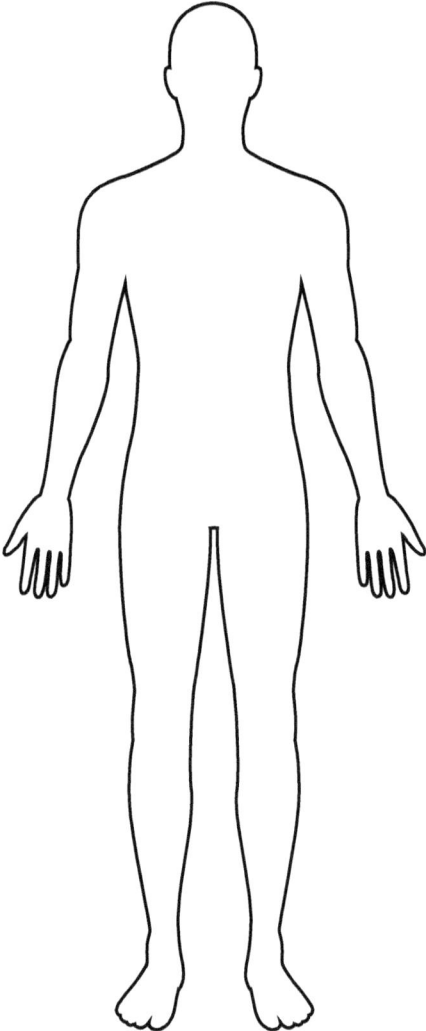

Quick Guide: Pain Locations

As seen in *The Everyday Pain Guide—Fix the Fire Damage*

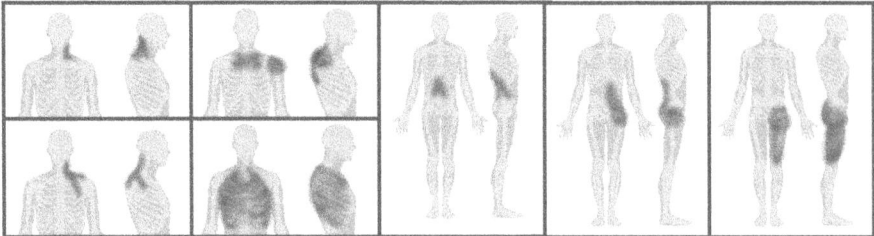

HOW MUCH PAIN TODAY?

Circle the face that best expresses your discomfort:

Wong-Baker FACES® Pain Rating Scale

0	2	4	6	8	10
No Pain	A Little Pain	A Little More Pain	Even More Pain	A Whole Lot Of Pain	Worst Pain

Notes:

_____

_____

_____

_____

_____

_____

_____

Remember to check out the Reinforce phases of body chemistry and stress biology action plans.

Notes:

_____

_____

_____

_____

_____

_____

_____

_____

_____

_____

_____

_____

_____

_____

_____

Reinforce
Activities

Week Two

REINFORCE – DAY 1

TODAY'S DATE: _____

Pick up to three of the following REINFORCE activities:

(Go to the Exercise Index in the Resources section at the back of the book, *Fix the Fire Damage*, to help you find these activities.)

☐ Plank hover (intermediate)

☐ Plank hover (advanced)

☐ Plank hover with inflate/deflate repetitions (advanced)

☐ Side plank (advanced)

☐ Downward dog with upward gaze (advanced)

☐ Neck turn and head nod

☐ Superman isometrics with neck focus

☐ Superman isometrics

☐ Tiny arm circles

☐ External shoulder rotation – repetitions + resistance (lying down)

☐ External shoulder rotation – repetitions + resistance (standing)

☐ Triceps extension pulldowns – repetitions + resistance

☐ Reach for the ceiling – repetitions + resistance

☐ Arm shoulder circles (forward rotation)

☐ Bent over fly

☐ Bench press with extra push

☐ Monster walk

☐ Clamshell pulse

☐ Reverse roman chair repetitions

☐ Dead bug – beginner

☐ Dead bug – intermediate

☐ Forearm plank – marching

☐ Bird dog

☐ Squat with side kick

☐ Ball-wall hip stability

☐ Supine hip circles – knee bent

☐ Supine hip circles – straight leg

REINFORCE ACTIVITIES

REINFORCE Activity #1: _____

Better? _____   Worse? _____   Same? _____

Other: _____

Notes: _____

_____

REINFORCE Activity #2: _____

Better? _____   Worse? _____   Same? _____

Other: _____

Notes: _____

_____

REINFORCE Activity #3: _____

Better? _____   Worse? _____   Same? _____

Other: _____

Notes: _____

_____

PAIN LOCATION:

Use this figure to color or shade-in the area of your pain however you like.

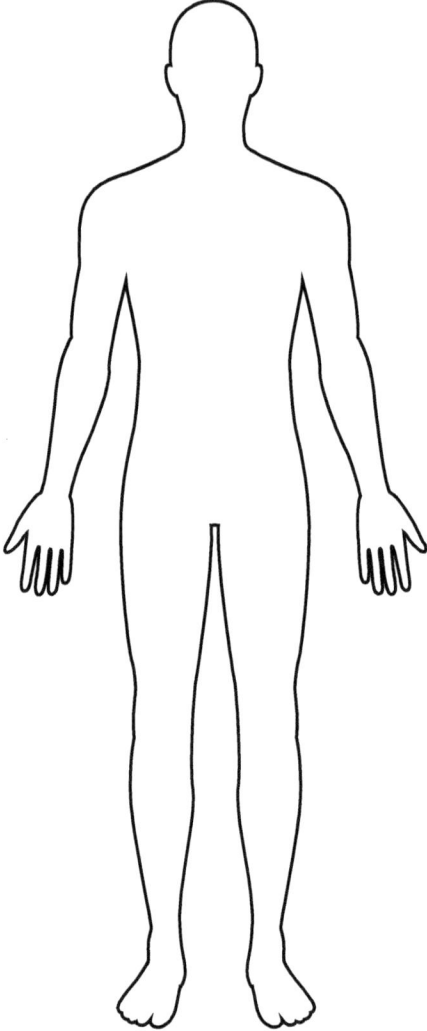

Quick Guide: Pain Locations

As seen in *The Everyday Pain Guide—Fix the Fire Damage*

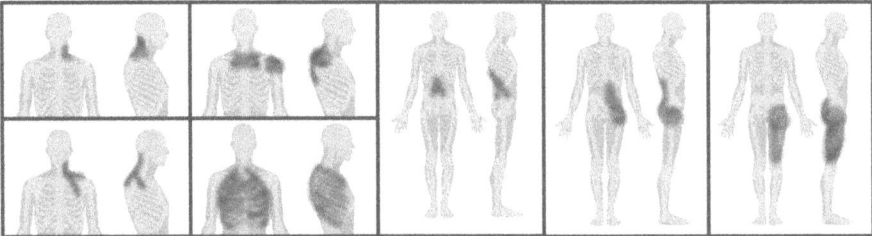

HOW MUCH PAIN TODAY?

Circle the face that best expresses your discomfort:

Wong-Baker FACES® Pain Rating Scale

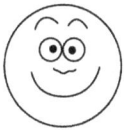 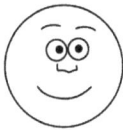 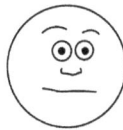 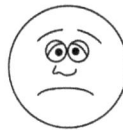 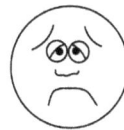 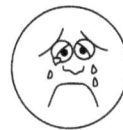

0	2	4	6	8	10
No Pain	A Little Pain	A Little More Pain	Even More Pain	A Whole Lot Of Pain	Worst Pain

Notes:

_____

_____

_____

_____

_____

_____

_____

_____

Remember to check out the Reinforce phases of body chemistry and stress biology action plans.

REINFORCE - DAY 2

TODAY'S DATE: _____

Pick up to three of the following REINFORCE activities:

(Go to the Exercise Index in the Resources section at the back of the book, *Fix the Fire Damage*, to help you find these activities.)

- [ ] Plank hover (intermediate)
- [ ] Plank hover (advanced)
- [ ] Plank hover with inflate/deflate repetitions (advanced)
- [ ] Side plank (advanced)
- [ ] Downward dog with upward gaze (advanced)
- [ ] Neck turn and head nod
- [ ] Superman isometrics with neck focus
- [ ] Superman isometrics
- [ ] Tiny arm circles
- [ ] External shoulder rotation – repetitions + resistance (lying down)
- [ ] External shoulder rotation – repetitions + resistance (standing)
- [ ] Triceps extension pulldowns – repetitions + resistance
- [ ] Reach for the ceiling – repetitions + resistance
- [ ] Arm shoulder circles (forward rotation)

- [ ] Bent over fly
- [ ] Bench press with extra push
- [ ] Monster walk
- [ ] Clamshell pulse
- [ ] Reverse roman chair repetitions
- [ ] Dead bug – beginner
- [ ] Dead bug – intermediate
- [ ] Forearm plank – marching
- [ ] Bird dog
- [ ] Squat with side kick
- [ ] Ball-wall hip stability
- [ ] Supine hip circles – knee bent
- [ ] Supine hip circles – straight leg

REINFORCE ACTIVITIES

REINFORCE Activity #1: _____

Better? _____   Worse? _____   Same? _____

Other: _____

Notes: _____

_____

REINFORCE Activity #2: _____

Better? _____   Worse? _____   Same? _____

Other: _____

Notes: _____

_____

REINFORCE Activity #3: _____

Better? _____   Worse? _____   Same? _____

Other: _____

Notes: _____

_____

PAIN LOCATION:

Use this figure to color or shade-in the area of your pain however you like.

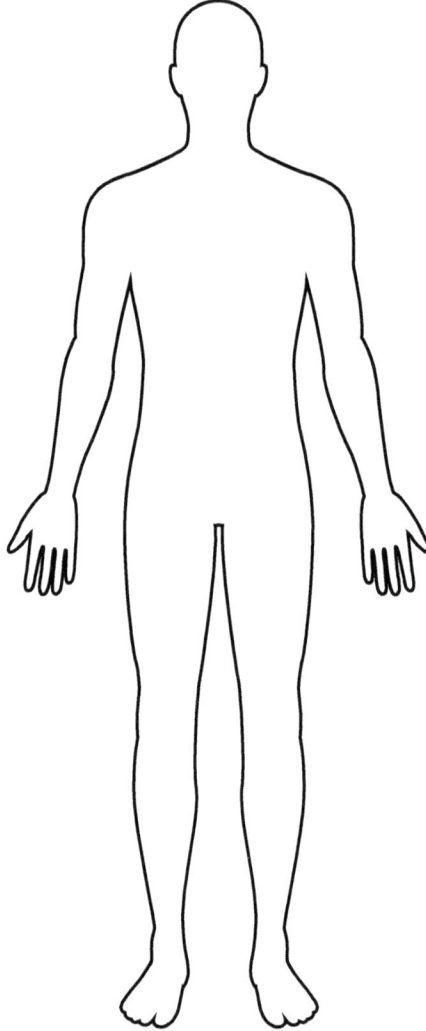

Quick Guide: Pain Locations

As seen in *The Everyday Pain Guide—Fix the Fire Damage*

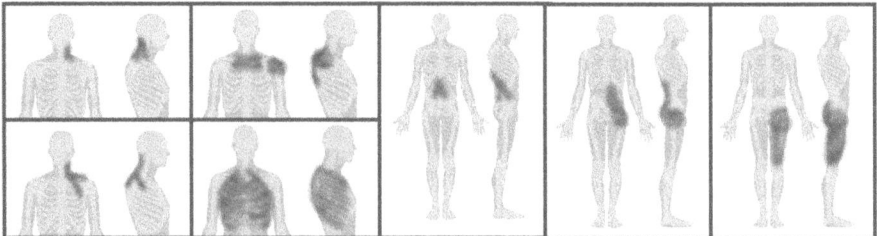

HOW MUCH PAIN TODAY?

Circle the face that best expresses your discomfort:

Wong-Baker FACES® Pain Rating Scale

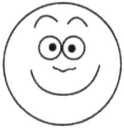 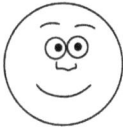 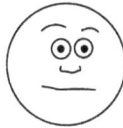 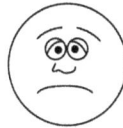 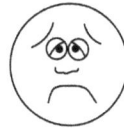 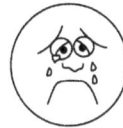

0	**2**	**4**	**6**	**8**	**10**
No Pain	A Little Pain	A Little More Pain	Even More Pain	A Whole Lot Of Pain	Worst Pain

Notes:

_____

_____

_____

_____

_____

_____

_____

Remember to check out the Reinforce phases of body chemistry and stress biology action plans.

REINFORCE – DAY 3

TODAY'S DATE: _____

Pick up to three of the following REINFORCE activities:

(Go to the Exercise Index in the Resources section at the back of the book, *Fix the Fire Damage*, to help you find these activities.)

- [ ] Plank hover (intermediate)
- [ ] Plank hover (advanced)
- [ ] Plank hover with inflate/deflate repetitions (advanced)
- [ ] Side plank (advanced)
- [ ] Downward dog with upward gaze (advanced)
- [ ] Neck turn and head nod
- [ ] Superman isometrics with neck focus
- [ ] Superman isometrics
- [ ] Tiny arm circles
- [ ] External shoulder rotation – repetitions + resistance (lying down)
- [ ] External shoulder rotation – repetitions + resistance (standing)
- [ ] Triceps extension pulldowns – repetitions + resistance
- [ ] Reach for the ceiling – repetitions + resistance
- [ ] Arm shoulder circles (forward rotation)

- [ ] Bent over fly
- [ ] Bench press with extra push
- [ ] Monster walk
- [ ] Clamshell pulse
- [ ] Reverse roman chair repetitions
- [ ] Dead bug – beginner
- [ ] Dead bug – intermediate
- [ ] Forearm plank – marching
- [ ] Bird dog
- [ ] Squat with side kick
- [ ] Ball-wall hip stability
- [ ] Supine hip circles – knee bent
- [ ] Supine hip circles – straight leg

REINFORCE ACTIVITIES

REINFORCE Activity #1: _____

Better? _____   Worse? _____   Same? _____

Other: _____

Notes: _____

_____

REINFORCE Activity #2: _____

Better? _____   Worse? _____   Same? _____

Other: _____

Notes: _____

_____

REINFORCE Activity #3: _____

Better? _____   Worse? _____   Same? _____

Other: _____

Notes: _____

_____

PAIN LOCATION:

Use this figure to color or shade-in the area of your pain however you like.

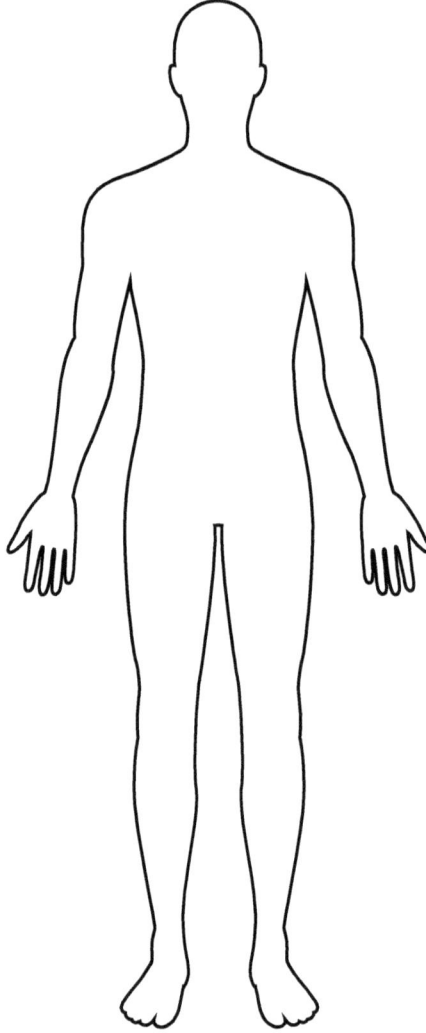

Quick Guide: Pain Locations

As seen in *The Everyday Pain Guide—Fix the Fire Damage*

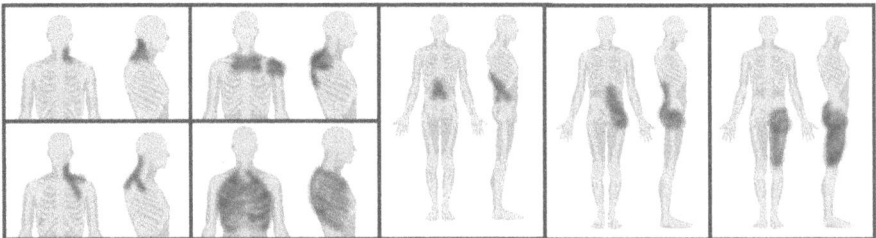

HOW MUCH PAIN TODAY?

Circle the face that best expresses your discomfort:

Wong-Baker FACES® Pain Rating Scale

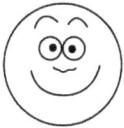 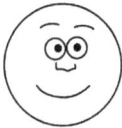 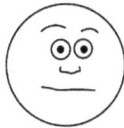 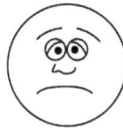 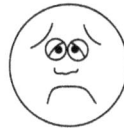 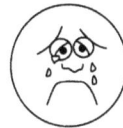

0	2	4	6	8	10
No Pain	A Little Pain	A Little More Pain	Even More Pain	A Whole Lot Of Pain	Worst Pain

Notes:

_____

_____

_____

_____

_____

_____

_____

Remember to check out the Reinforce phases of body chemistry and stress biology action plans.

REINFORCE – DAY 4

TODAY'S DATE: _____

Pick up to three of the following REINFORCE activities:

(Go to the Exercise Index in the Resources section at the back of the book, *Fix the Fire Damage*, to help you find these activities.)

☐ Plank hover (intermediate)

☐ Plank hover (advanced)

☐ Plank hover with inflate/deflate repetitions (advanced)

☐ Side plank (advanced)

☐ Downward dog with upward gaze (advanced)

☐ Neck turn and head nod

☐ Superman isometrics with neck focus

☐ Superman isometrics

☐ Tiny arm circles

☐ External shoulder rotation – repetitions + resistance (lying down)

☐ External shoulder rotation – repetitions + resistance (standing)

☐ Triceps extension pulldowns – repetitions + resistance

☐ Reach for the ceiling – repetitions + resistance

☐ Arm shoulder circles (forward rotation)

☐ Bent over fly

☐ Bench press with extra push

☐ Monster walk

☐ Clamshell pulse

☐ Reverse roman chair repetitions

☐ Dead bug – beginner

☐ Dead bug – intermediate

☐ Forearm plank – marching

☐ Bird dog

☐ Squat with side kick

☐ Ball-wall hip stability

☐ Supine hip circles – knee bent

☐ Supine hip circles – straight leg

REINFORCE ACTIVITIES

REINFORCE Activity #1: _____

Better? _____   Worse? _____   Same? _____

Other: _____

Notes: _____

_____

REINFORCE Activity #2: _____

Better? _____   Worse? _____   Same? _____

Other: _____

Notes: _____

_____

REINFORCE Activity #3: _____

Better? _____   Worse? _____   Same? _____

Other: _____

Notes: _____

_____

PAIN LOCATION:

Use this figure to color or shade-in the area of your pain however you like.

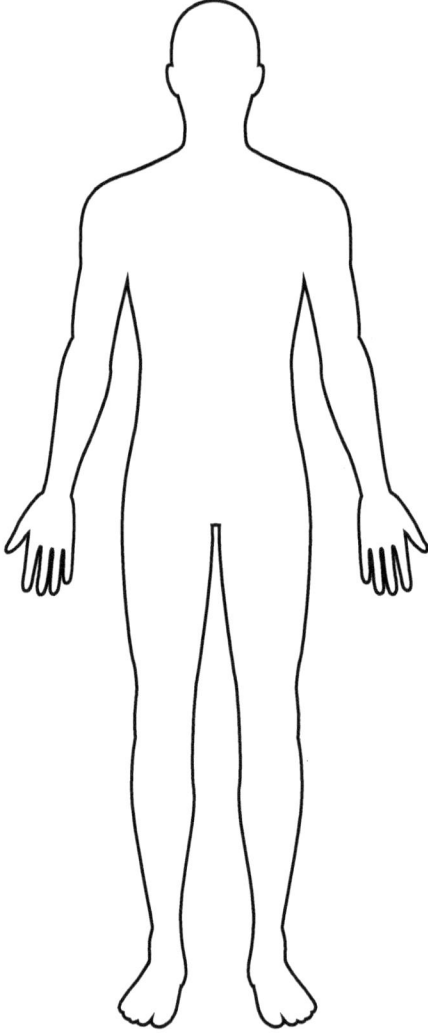

Quick Guide: Pain Locations

As seen in *The Everyday Pain Guide—Fix the Fire Damage*

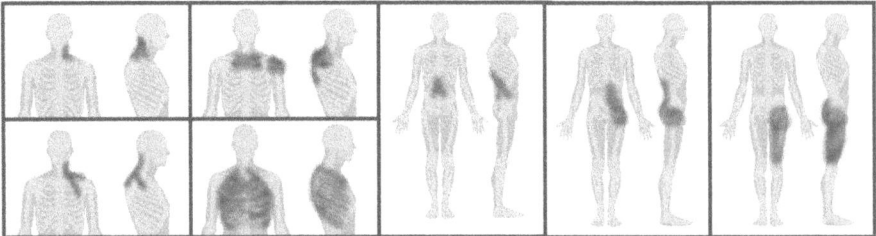

HOW MUCH PAIN TODAY?

Circle the face that best expresses your discomfort:

Wong-Baker FACES® Pain Rating Scale

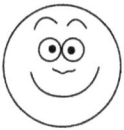 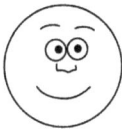 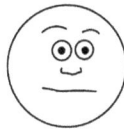 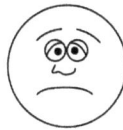 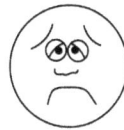 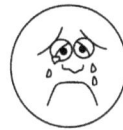

0	2	4	6	8	10
No Pain	A Little Pain	A Little More Pain	Even More Pain	A Whole Lot Of Pain	Worst Pain

Notes:

_____

_____

_____

_____

_____

_____

_____

Remember to check out the Reinforce phases of body chemistry and stress biology action plans.

TODAY'S DATE: _____

Pick up to three of the following REINFORCE activities:

(Go to the Exercise Index in the Resources section at the back of the book, *Fix the Fire Damage*, to help you find these activities.)

☐ Plank hover (intermediate)

☐ Plank hover (advanced)

☐ Plank hover with inflate/deflate repetitions (advanced)

☐ Side plank (advanced)

☐ Downward dog with upward gaze (advanced)

☐ Neck turn and head nod

☐ Superman isometrics with neck focus

☐ Superman isometrics

☐ Tiny arm circles

☐ External shoulder rotation – repetitions + resistance (lying down)

☐ External shoulder rotation – repetitions + resistance (standing)

☐ Triceps extension pulldowns – repetitions + resistance

☐ Reach for the ceiling – repetitions + resistance

☐ Arm shoulder circles (forward rotation)

☐ Bent over fly

☐ Bench press with extra push

☐ Monster walk

☐ Clamshell pulse

☐ Reverse roman chair repetitions

☐ Dead bug – beginner

☐ Dead bug – intermediate

☐ Forearm plank – marching

☐ Bird dog

☐ Squat with side kick

☐ Ball-wall hip stability

☐ Supine hip circles – knee bent

☐ Supine hip circles – straight leg

REINFORCE ACTIVITIES

REINFORCE Activity #1: _____

Better? _____   Worse? _____   Same? _____

Other: _____

Notes: _____

_____

REINFORCE Activity #2: _____

Better? _____   Worse? _____   Same? _____

Other: _____

Notes: _____

_____

REINFORCE Activity #3: _____

Better? _____   Worse? _____   Same? _____

Other: _____

Notes: _____

_____

PAIN LOCATION:

Use this figure to color or shade-in the area of your pain however you like.

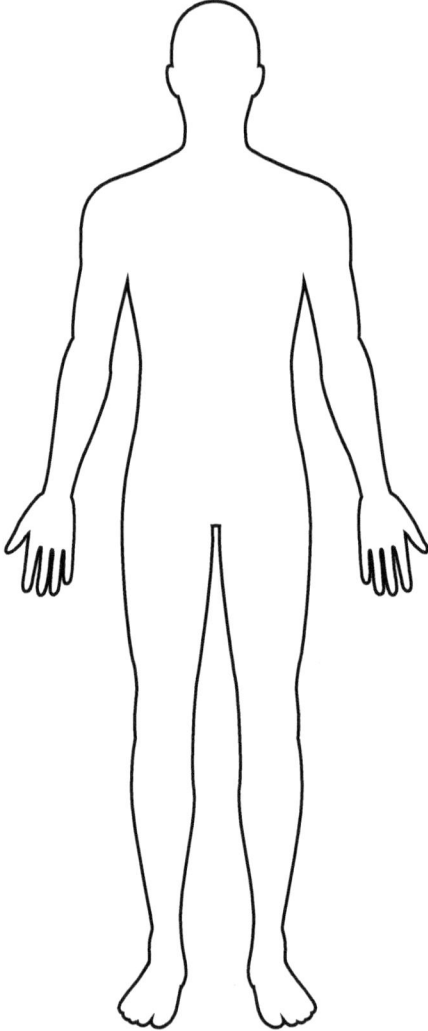

Quick Guide: Pain Locations

As seen in *The Everyday Pain Guide—Fix the Fire Damage*

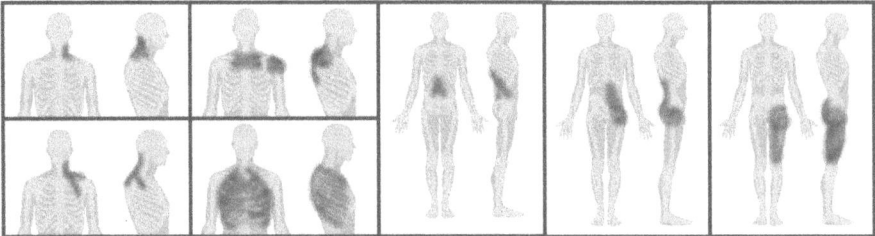

HOW MUCH PAIN TODAY?

Circle the face that best expresses your discomfort:

Wong-Baker FACES® Pain Rating Scale

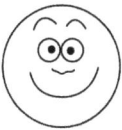 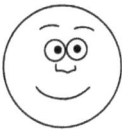 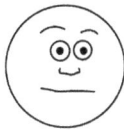 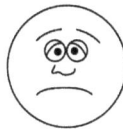 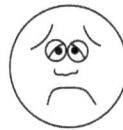 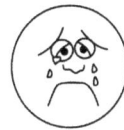

0	2	4	6	8	10
No Pain	A Little Pain	A Little More Pain	Even More Pain	A Whole Lot Of Pain	Worst Pain

Notes:

_____

_____

_____

_____

_____

_____

_____

Remember to check out the Reinforce phases of body chemistry and stress biology action plans.

REINFORCE – DAY 6

TODAY'S DATE: _____

Pick up to three of the following REINFORCE activities:

(Go to the Exercise Index in the Resources section at the back of the book, *Fix the Fire Damage*, to help you find these activities.)

☐ Plank hover (intermediate)

☐ Plank hover (advanced)

☐ Plank hover with inflate/deflate repetitions (advanced)

☐ Side plank (advanced)

☐ Downward dog with upward gaze (advanced)

☐ Neck turn and head nod

☐ Superman isometrics with neck focus

☐ Superman isometrics

☐ Tiny arm circles

☐ External shoulder rotation – repetitions + resistance (lying down)

☐ External shoulder rotation – repetitions + resistance (standing)

☐ Triceps extension pulldowns – repetitions + resistance

☐ Reach for the ceiling – repetitions + resistance

☐ Arm shoulder circles (forward rotation)

☐ Bent over fly

☐ Bench press with extra push

☐ Monster walk

☐ Clamshell pulse

☐ Reverse roman chair repetitions

☐ Dead bug – beginner

☐ Dead bug – intermediate

☐ Forearm plank – marching

☐ Bird dog

☐ Squat with side kick

☐ Ball-wall hip stability

☐ Supine hip circles – knee bent

☐ Supine hip circles – straight leg

REINFORCE ACTIVITIES

REINFORCE Activity #1: _____

Better? _____   Worse? _____   Same? _____

Other: _____

Notes: _____

_____

REINFORCE Activity #2: _____

Better? _____   Worse? _____   Same? _____

Other: _____

Notes: _____

_____

REINFORCE Activity #3: _____

Better? _____   Worse? _____   Same? _____

Other: _____

Notes: _____

_____

PAIN LOCATION:

Use this figure to color or shade-in the area of your pain however you like.

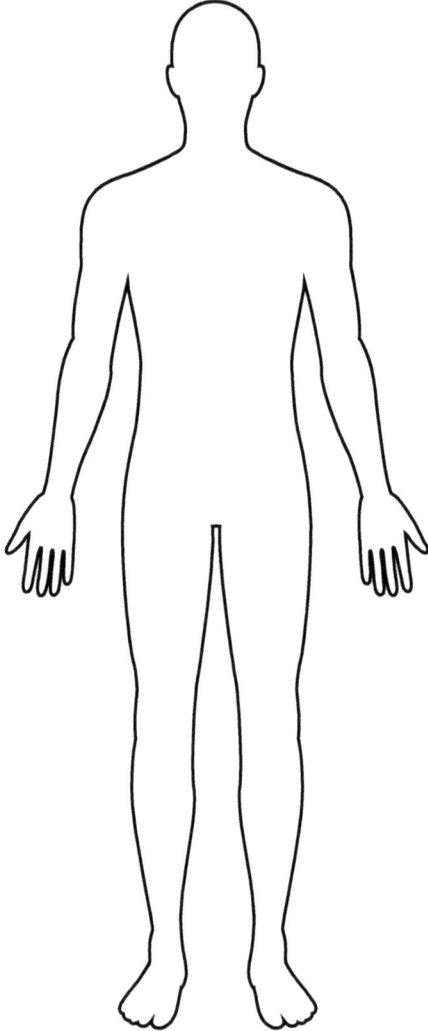

Quick Guide: Pain Locations

As seen in *The Everyday Pain Guide—Fix the Fire Damage*

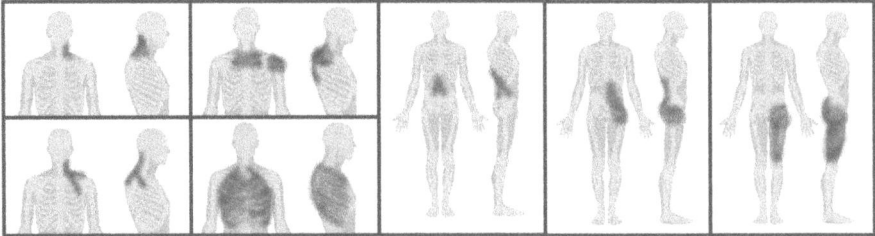

HOW MUCH PAIN TODAY?

Circle the face that best expresses your discomfort:

Wong-Baker FACES® Pain Rating Scale

0	2	4	6	8	10
No Pain	A Little Pain	A Little More Pain	Even More Pain	A Whole Lot Of Pain	Worst Pain

Notes:

_____

_____

_____

_____

_____

_____

_____

Remember to check out the Reinforce phases of body chemistry and stress biology action plans.

TODAY'S DATE: _____

Pick up to three of the following REINFORCE activities:

(Go to the Exercise Index in the Resources section at the back of the book, *Fix the Fire Damage*, to help you find these activities.)

- ☐ Plank hover (intermediate)
- ☐ Plank hover (advanced)
- ☐ Plank hover with inflate/deflate repetitions (advanced)
- ☐ Side plank (advanced)
- ☐ Downward dog with upward gaze (advanced)
- ☐ Neck turn and head nod
- ☐ Superman isometrics with neck focus
- ☐ Superman isometrics
- ☐ Tiny arm circles
- ☐ External shoulder rotation – repetitions + resistance (lying down)
- ☐ External shoulder rotation – repetitions + resistance (standing)
- ☐ Triceps extension pulldowns – repetitions + resistance
- ☐ Reach for the ceiling – repetitions + resistance
- ☐ Arm shoulder circles (forward rotation)

- ☐ Bent over fly
- ☐ Bench press with extra push
- ☐ Monster walk
- ☐ Clamshell pulse
- ☐ Reverse roman chair repetitions
- ☐ Dead bug – beginner
- ☐ Dead bug – intermediate
- ☐ Forearm plank – marching
- ☐ Bird dog
- ☐ Squat with side kick
- ☐ Ball-wall hip stability
- ☐ Supine hip circles – knee bent
- ☐ Supine hip circles – straight leg

REINFORCE ACTIVITIES

REINFORCE Activity #1: _____

Better? _____   Worse? _____   Same? _____

Other: _____

Notes: _____

_____

REINFORCE Activity #2: _____

Better? _____   Worse? _____   Same? _____

Other: _____

Notes: _____

_____

REINFORCE Activity #3: _____

Better? _____   Worse? _____   Same? _____

Other: _____

Notes: _____

_____

PAIN LOCATION:

Use this figure to color or shade-in the area of your pain however you like.

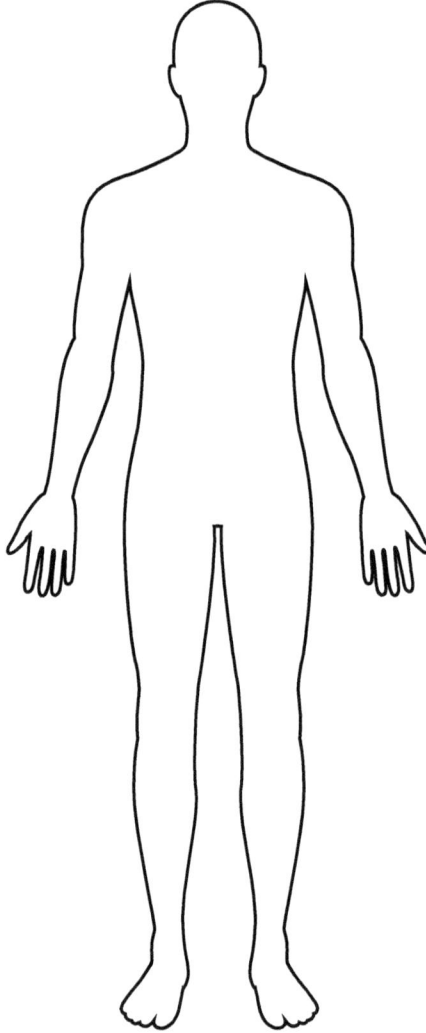

Quick Guide: Pain Locations

As seen in *The Everyday Pain Guide—Fix the Fire Damage*

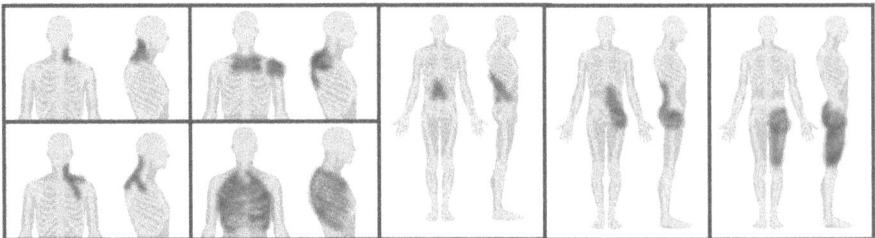

HOW MUCH PAIN TODAY?

Circle the face that best expresses your discomfort:

Wong-Baker FACES® Pain Rating Scale

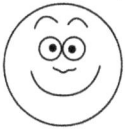 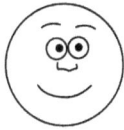 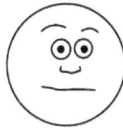 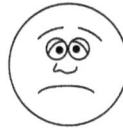 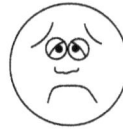 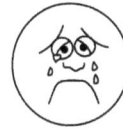

0	2	4	6	8	10
No Pain	A Little Pain	A Little More Pain	Even More Pain	A Whole Lot Of Pain	Worst Pain

Notes:

_____

_____

_____

_____

_____

_____

_____

Remember to check out the Reinforce phases of body chemistry and stress biology action plans.

My Everyday Pain Story

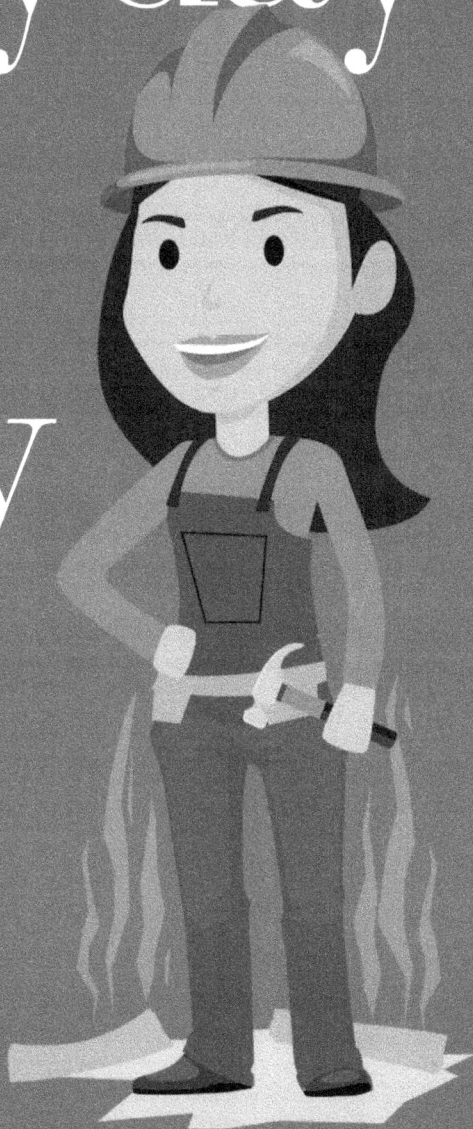

My Everyday Pain Story

When I release my pain, I...

_____

_____

_____

_____

_____

_____

_____

_____

_____

_____

_____

My Everyday Pain Story

When I have less pain, I look forward to...
doing/feeling/being:

_____

_____

_____

_____

_____

_____

_____

_____

_____

_____

_____

My Everyday Pain Story

When I am stronger, I look forward to...
doing/feeling/being:

_____

_____

_____

_____

_____

_____

_____

_____

_____

_____

_____

_____

My Everyday Pain Story

When I am more grounded in my body, I look forward to...doing/feeling/being:

_____

_____

_____

_____

_____

_____

_____

_____

_____

_____

My Everyday Pain Story

My first or most memorable pain
experience or injury as a child

_____

_____

_____

_____

_____

_____

_____

_____

_____

_____

What part of me was hurt?

How did it happen?

Who was there with me or was I alone?

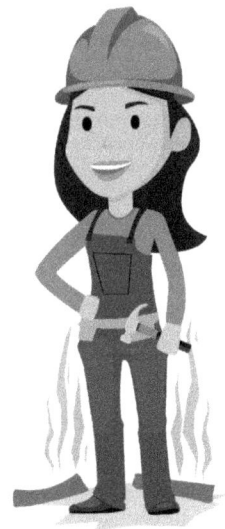

My Everyday Pain Story

If there was a parent, guardian, friend or teacher nearby, how did they react to my injury?

If I was alone at the time, how did I feel about that?

Were any of these feelings present: shame, blame, anger, fear, embarrassment, humor, achievement?

Notes:

_____

_____

_____

_____

_____

_____

_____

_____

_____

_____

_____

_____

_____

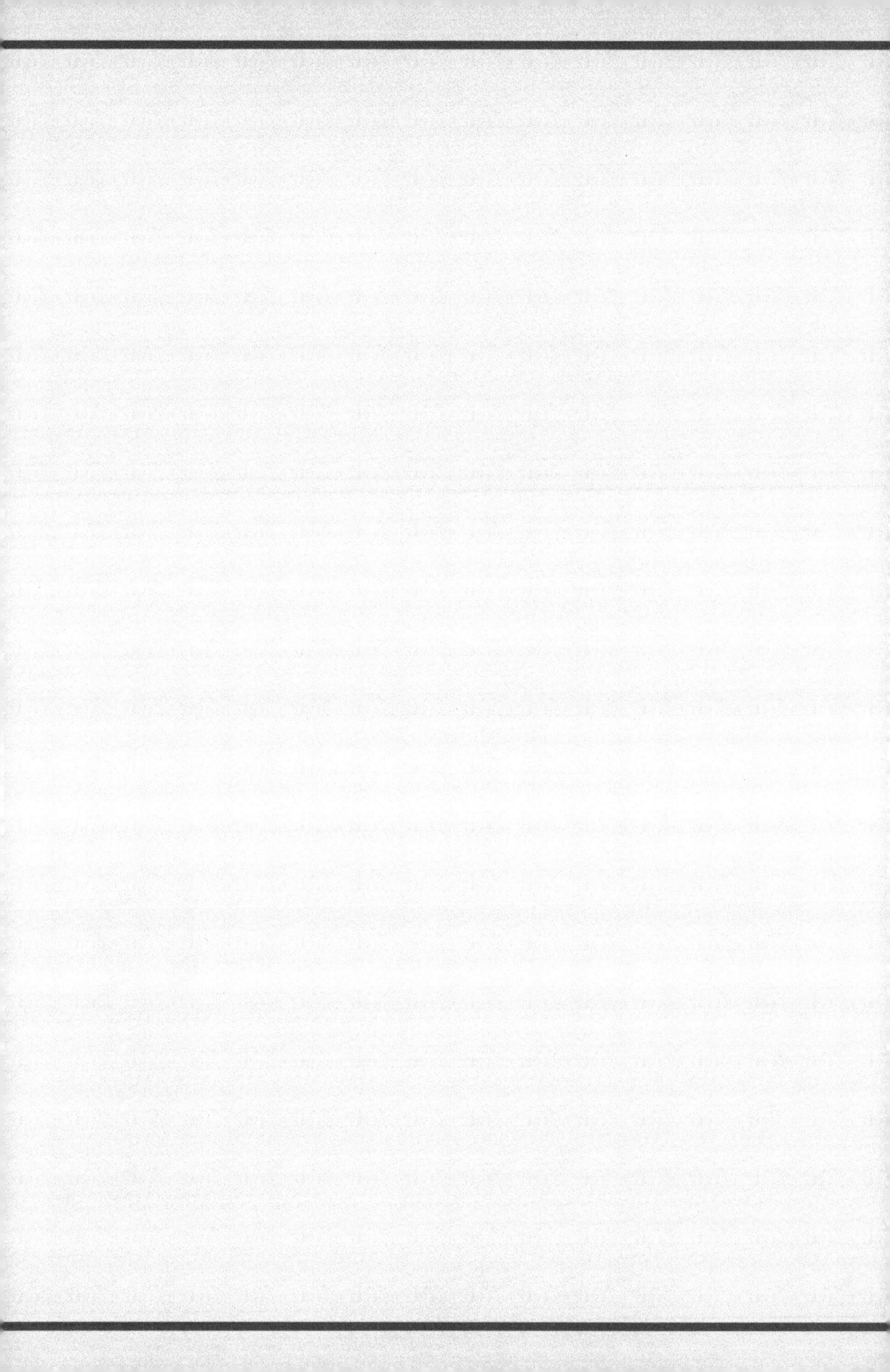

What
the
Pros
Say

A Question and Answer
Session with the Pros

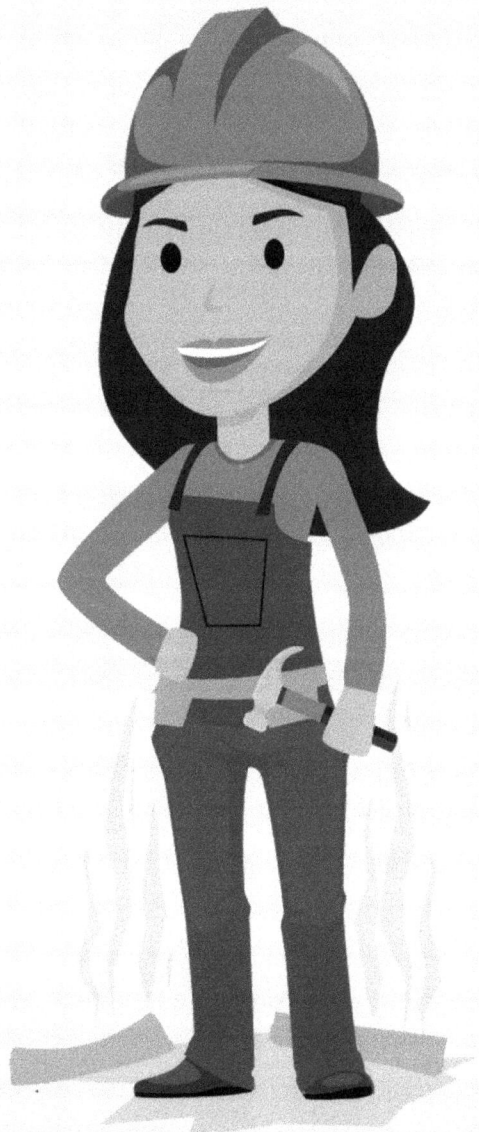

WHAT THE PROS SAY

NOW THAT YOU'VE TAKEN YOURSELF FROM the "five alarm fire" kind of pain down to a manageable situation and mostly pain free, please stay mindful. You're not done. The next and equally important part of the process is to continue with the Reinforce stage of your 3-pronged Stop Everyday Pain approach. You've gained some tools to begin the reinforcing process in the Actions Steps section, but there's even better quality of life available to you. Your body is designed to be much stronger and more agile than it has been to this point, even if you thought you were just fine before the pain experience. You may consider yourself to be a well-conditioned athlete, but if you've been taken by surprise with a bout of everyday pain, then the conditioning you've had to date, while valuable, might not be relevant to the demands of your day-to-day life. Everyone can use some serious fine-tuning from time to time.

It's at this stage, when people feel better, that they take their eye off the ball. However, when you let your guard down, you make room for the pain to come back. Keeping your guard up does not mean you continue to be anxious or tentative about movements or activities, constantly worried that pain *might* come back. Instead, it means you now persist in returning to the selective activities that you have learned *will* support and reinforce your body against future pain. You are now equipped with better information about what your body's specific needs are and you are willing to respect those. With the refined knowledge gained by working through the Body Mechanics Repair Guide and Action Plan during your recent pain experience, you can now engage fully in all your usual movements and activities again without pain. To avoid relapse, however, you must also *continue* to incorporate this new toolkit.

In my chiropractic practice, the next step for patients is to get connected with integrative and adjunctive therapies. It's time to build on your progress by tapping into the larger healthcare and wellness community.

What follows next is an exploration of a few different types of providers known for dealing with body mechanics. The perspectives shared are from six different professionals spanning three different disciplines as they touch on their approach to treating pain, specifically from a *mechanical* point of view. These six voices are practitioners local to Seattle, Washington, who kindly responded to my request for contributions to this book series. I urge you to use some of the questions addressed here as a jumping off point while you consider your next phase in the pain repair process.

Please note that none of this is necessarily an endorsement for or against a specific modality or method or provider. This section aims primarily to show you a peek at what else is out there. While each response was unique, there are a few common threads that you might also detect as you read through them. At the end, I'll give you a little bit of my take on it.

Y. L.

MEET THE PROS

Dr. Einat Arian, PhD, ND

www.gentlehealingarts.com

Dr. Arian is a naturopathic physician who holds a Diplomate in Craniosacral Therapy from the Integrative Bodywork Institute. Her first doctorate was in the field of neurophysiology from Hebrew University in Jerusalem in 1997. In her Seattle practice, she has found her niche within post-concussion syndrome and pediatrics.

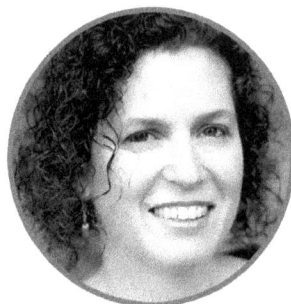

Susanne Michaud, DPT

www.strideseattle.com

Physical therapist and owner of Stride Physio, Susanne is passionate about anatomy, alignment and beautiful movement. As a lifelong learner and constant runner, Susanne draws from a deep toolbox of skill, experience and empathy to restore and improve people's movement and facilitate living life to the fullest. Susanne specializes in orthopedics, sports and manual therapy. She has special interest in pain science, return-to-running programs, custom foot orthoses, posture restoration, aging athletes, musical performance, autoimmune conditions, cancer care, bike fits and ergonomics. She thrives

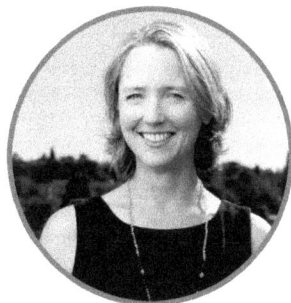

on figuring out the mechanics behind movement dysfunction and is tenacious about finding the right program for returning people to mobility, independence and joyful movement. She received her doctorate in physical therapy from the University of Washington, School of Medicine.

Richelle Ricard, LMT
www.yogaengineer.com

Richelle has worked with bodies for over 30 years. Her unique perspective on pain, posture and movement comes from her eclectic collection of experience in all of the following: sports medicine, clinical massage, yoga and movement therapy, energetic bodywork, rehabilitation medicine and education. When she's not teaching somewhere around the world, sharing the wisdom of the physical body with yoga teachers and students, you can find her in Portland, OR offering bodywork sessions and leading weekly yoga classes and workshops. She is the author of the book *The Yoga Engineer's Manual*.

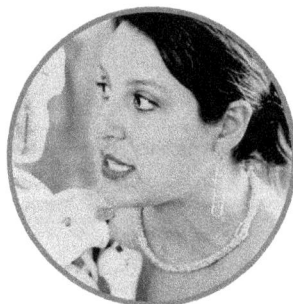

Heidi Gans, PT
www.heidiganspt.com

Heidi received her master's degree in physical therapy from Duke University in 1997 and has been practicing physical therapy ever since. She started out treating patients recovering from trauma and significant neurological disorders at Seattle's Harborview Medical Center. Subsequently, she worked with dancers, runners, skiers, and triathletes in sports medicine settings. Currently, her practice serves varied physical therapy needs from joint injuries to back pain, postural issues to strains and sprains as well as biomechanical issues to muscle

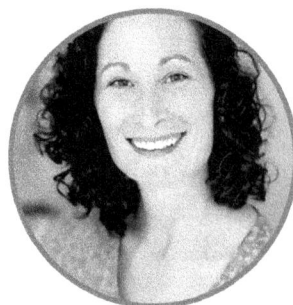

imbalance. She is also teaching anatomy workshops in the Seattle area and movement education at Cornish College of the Arts.

Part of what informs her professional practice is her experience as a dancer with the New York City Ballet, performing at Lincoln Center and touring internationally. During these years, Heidi worked with world-renowned choreographers and musicians and danced alongside some of the greatest movers on Earth. This life as a dancer gave her firsthand experience with many injuries and taught her how to avoid, manage and recover from many of them. It also left her with a lifelong appreciation for the fruits of diligence, hard work, strength and flexibility, which continue to inform her work and lifestyle.

Michaelle Edwards

www.yogalign.com

Michaelle Edwards is a licensed massage therapist, posture and movement educator, author and musician located in Kauai, Hawaii. She is the creator of YogAlign and FitAlign Posture Trainings which are specifically designed to provide people of all ages with safe and comfortable tools for optimal spine alignment. Michaelle has been teaching breath-based alignment techniques for over three decades, and she conducts seminars and trainings all over the globe. She is a writer for the *Huffington Post* and is the author of numerous articles on posture and the book *YogAlign: Pain-Free Yoga from Your Inner Core*.

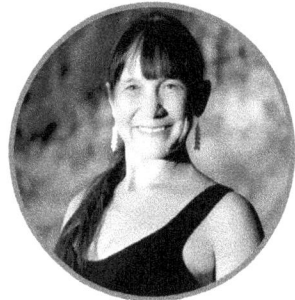

Liz Durkin, OT

www.irgpt.com/staff/elizabeth-durkin

Liz Durkin has more than 15 years of professional experience practicing a variety of alternative healing modalities including Traditional Chinese Medicine, Therapeutic Massage, Reiki, and Acutonics® (sound/vibrational healing). At the root of her practice is a belief in the body's innate wisdom and ability to heal itself when reconnected to nature. She is passionate about supporting people on their journeys back to health and uses her knowledge of body and its energetic pathways to encourage wellbeing and being well. After 15 years of practicing Eastern medicine, Liz decided to return to graduate school to study Western medicine and deepen her commitment to integrating the two. She received a Master of Occupational Therapy from the University of Washington in 2015, where she met Kelly Clancy, whose like-minded teachings struck a deep, resonant chord. Kelly invited her to practice at the Seattle Center for Structural Medicine in September 2016 when she also began training at the Northwest School of Structural Medicine. In 2017, Liz was certified as a Bowen Therapist and Level 1 Tensegrity Medicine[1] Practitioner, combining all of her skills into a practice that addresses musculoskeletal disorders, chronic pain, and autoimmune disorders with a unique holistic approach.

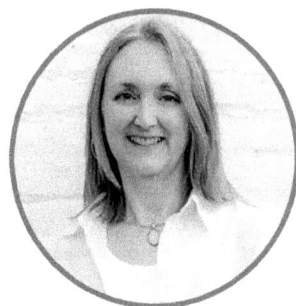

---

1. "tensegrity" is a term used in architecture defined as: the characteristic property of a stable three-dimensional structure consisting of members under tension that are contiguous and members under compression that are not. Tensegrity Medicine is a trademarked method of working with the body in a rehabilitative capacity.

ASK THE PROS

Ask the Pros

How would you describe your role to someone seeking help for chronic recurring aches and pains?

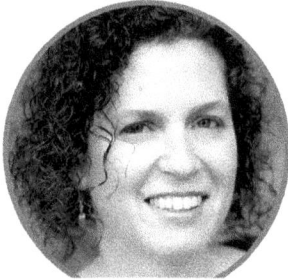

Einat Arian, PhD, ND

I try to help people believe that things can change, that they can be free of pain.

I also focus on finding physical restrictions around the nervous system and in the fascia matrix[2] that affect the entire system.

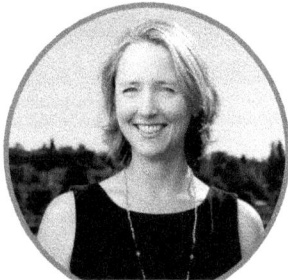

Susanne Michaud, DPT

My role is to guide someone in their darkness toward the light of understanding pain and, in that understanding, better manage and correct the physical perpetrators of that pain. Pain is not "one size fits all." As such, it is my role to truly understand a person's pain story and to help them rewrite that story to include the joy of moving.

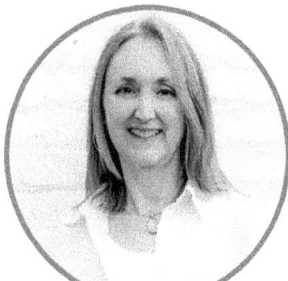

Liz Durkin, OT

I am a facilitator and someone who has been down a similar road. My role is to assist clients to look for and find the root (mind, body, spirit) of chronic recurring aches and pain through listening, reflecting, and using therapeutic use of self (sharing my own experiences). Together, we co-create a plan to meet each client's individual needs. I explain to clients that I am only assisting them to find ways to heal. I try to instill the understanding that healing comes from within and depends upon their ability/willingness to reconnect to the highest self/ nature/universe.

---

2. The "fascia matrix" refers to the network of connective tissue all over the body. There is scientific controversy about the significance of this as a distinct structure. You can read more about it with author Tom Myers of Anatomy Trains fame.

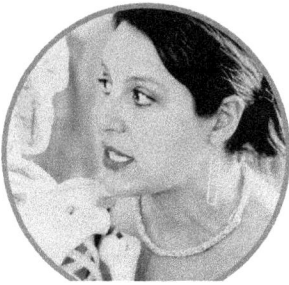

Richelle Ricard, LMT

My role is to observe the patterns of posture, movement and holding that sometimes we are no longer able to feel or observe in ourselves. Once identified, I work together with students and clients to unwind the physical and energetic (psycho-emotional or mind-based) roots of those patterns. Then we'll develop a plan of self-care and homework activities that support the hands-on work.

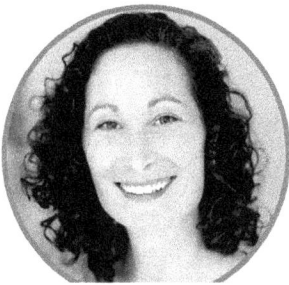

Heidi Gans, PT

My best role as a PT is as a "fellow explorer and guide." Pain is an interpretation we make in the brain to help us avoid danger. However, in chronic pain, we often lose our ability to determine which aspects of pain are protective and informative and which have simply become habitual and reactionary. My role is to help my clients gain more fine-tuned awareness and sensitivity regarding their experience of pain and then to guide them in "the direction of good."

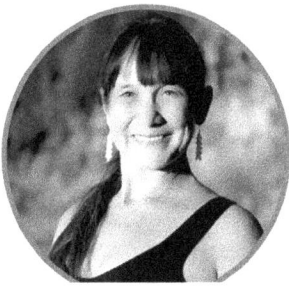

Michaelle Edwards

I am a posture educator who evaluates clients' posture and breathing habits. Postural alignment dysfunction is a major cause of chronic aches and pains, so I instruct clients to perform breathing and postural balancing techniques, which work at the neuromuscular level, recruiting the core trunk muscles to work primarily as stabilizers. I focus on habits of daily life including walking, sitting, standing and bending forward.

Ask the Pros

How do you feel about working with patients who are concurrently also receiving other care (acupuncture, massage, chiropractic, physical therapy, psychotherapy, other)? Do you find it affects outcomes positively or negatively?

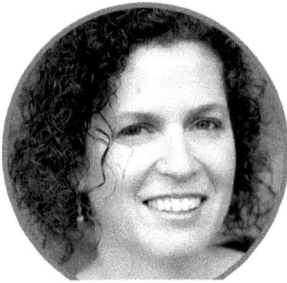

I love working with other professions and feel, in general, that we all contribute to the progress of the patient. I do prefer to work alongside practitioners who I know tend to think similarly to myself and use low-force techniques.

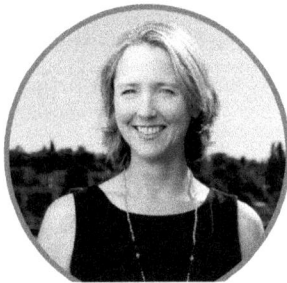

Einat Arian, PhD, ND

I'm a huge advocate of lifelong health maintenance, working on many dimensions of health. I strongly believe in working with all care providers whom the patient entrusts. I also believe it's important for open communication to occur between these providers so that a person is not "over" treated and does not get conflicting information that could stymie their success.

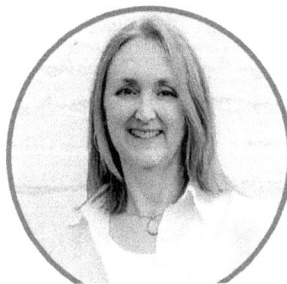

Susanne Michaud, DPT

I believe it does take a proverbial village to help someone with chronic pain. I support clients receiving other care but warn against over stimulating the nervous system with too much input because a) it makes it difficult to discern what is working and b) can trigger flare-ups of pain. Generally, I suggest that a client should not have more than one treatment session a day, and for some two days in between, which often works out positively.

Liz Durkin, OT

I think there is no single magic bullet for any condition. We are whole beings that exist on a spectrum of experiences. Bodywork such as what I provide has many benefits, but it is not the "end-all be-all." I believe deeply in a well-rounded approach to finding wellness. A team effort can have remarkably positive outcomes, especially when all members of the team understand their individual roles AND how they interact with the other treatments.

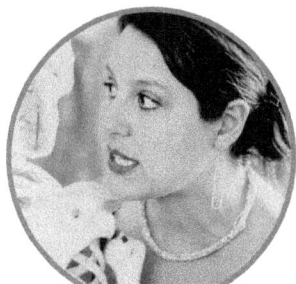

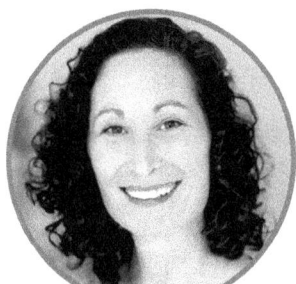

Richelle Ricard, LMT

Most of my clients are seeing or have seen multiple practitioners from other disciplines, and I always assume this is a positive thing. I feel a sense of community and collaboration with therapists and doctors who do good work and am grateful for their expertise. Sharing clients with other specialists allows me to focus on my tools and skill set and trust that others are doing the same so that together we are able to offer the best possible care.

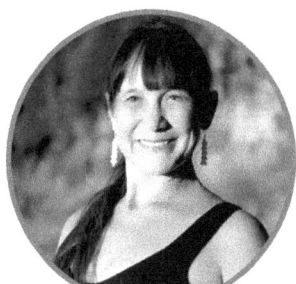

Heidi Gans, PT

Outcomes vary depending on the modality. Physical therapy or deep tissue massage sometimes seems to impede the progress for my clients—it depends. I do ask clients to show me all programmed exercises they are doing to make sure they are not doing ones that contribute to more pain.

I have seen dependence on bodywork that disables a person from taking the self-care steps needed to stabilize their spine or joints without this reliance on habitual passive treatments.

Michaelle Edwards

Ask the Pros

Do you counsel patients/clients about how to coordinate integrative care with other professionals? If so, what are your common recommendations?

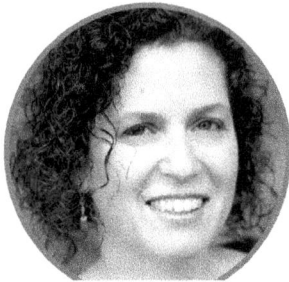

My main recommendation is not to try too many new things at once and to spread treatments out. I definitely do not recommend seeing two practitioners on the same day.

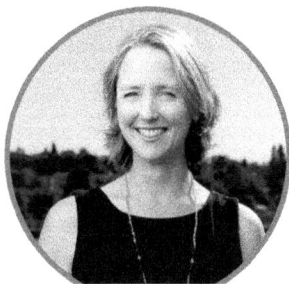

Einat Arian, PhD, ND

I have all patients sign a HIPAA release so that open communication is approved by the patient. I ask about the care they are receiving and if they would be okay with me writing notes or making phone calls to their other providers. I will make suggestions for other care providers if I see it would be of benefit and they are not currently receiving it. I always follow-up about appointments they've had with other practitioners and what they learned from those sessions in order to integrate that into my plan of care.

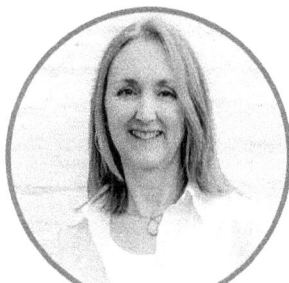

Susanne Michaud, DPT

Yes, our clinic uses a team approach, and I often refer clients out for nutritional, acupuncture (Japanese), naturopathic, and gentle chiropractic care (NUCCA, network, Atlas, myofascial). Our clinic has in-house movement specialists who utilize modalities such as MELT[3], Gyrotonic, neuro-fascial release and restorative yoga, but if other types of physical therapy are necessary, we also will refer out with specific recommendations.

Liz Durkin, OT

---

3. MELT stands for Myofascial Energetic Length Technique and was developed by a fitness trainer named Sue Hitzmann.

I do. Most often I recommend acupuncture, chiropractic, naturopathy and nutritional therapy. Psychotherapy is also something I recommend…I think we ALL need therapy on some level.

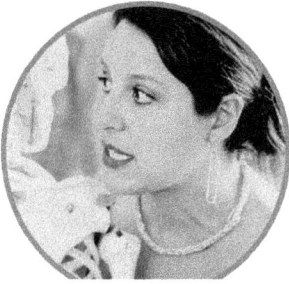

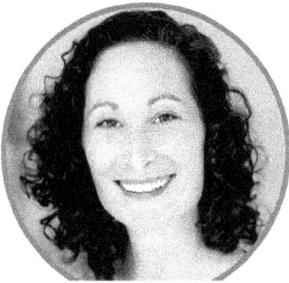

Richelle Ricard, LMT

My most consistent recommendation is to, whenever possible, allow at least 24 hours between sessions. This is to allow the nervous system to integrate the input from each session before introducing new information. I believe our bodies are much more sensitive and responsive than we realize, and allowing time for things to settle is both respectful and wise. I have also noticed that running from one therapy to the next can amp up the nervous system, which tends to be at odds with healing.

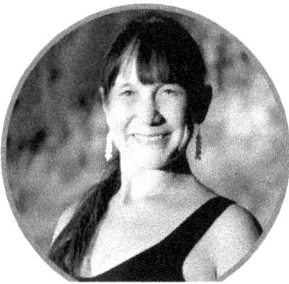

Heidi Gans, PT

Many clients see other professionals for massage, acupuncture or chiropractic; however, the ultimate goal is to be healthcare self-reliant.

Michaelle Edwards

Do you make lifestyle recommendations? If so, are there one or two that you recommend more often than others and why?

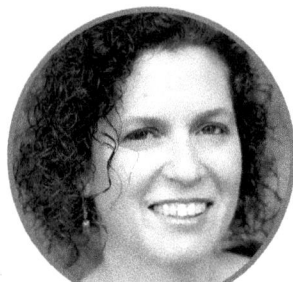

Supplements: Mg/Cal (reverse ratio) and/or Epsom salt bath. Fish oils (other omega-3), sometimes anti-inflammatories (like turmeric, Phytoprofen, or even ibuprofen).

Sleep: I sometimes recommend sleeping with a pillow between the knees if sleeping on the side, legs bent. And sleeping with a pillow under the knees when sleeping on the back if I suspect tight hip flexors or if people mention they wake up with body tension.

Einat Arian, PhD, ND

Yes, lifestyle recommendations are key. I often work with a person's sleep hygiene and bolstering (pillow positioning and support), on their home and office computer set-ups, querying them about drug and alcohol intake, any issues around sexual activity relating to pain or movement dysfunction, and of course general fitness engagement.

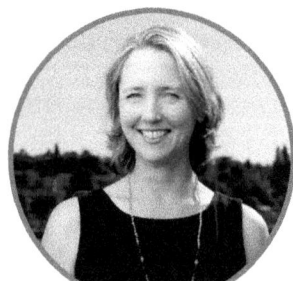

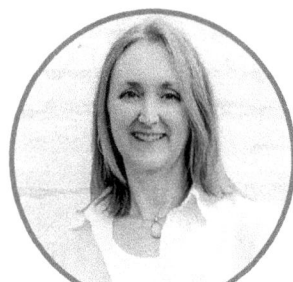

Susanne Michaud, DPT

In order of frequency, I'd say fitness, sleep, and work habits are what I talk about with people the most.

Yes: mindfulness, breathing and learning to tone the vagal nerve[4]. Inflammation cannot be healed within a sympathetic (fight, flight or freeze) state, so we discuss the benefit of techniques that stimulate a parasympathetic (relaxation) response. With some, I might discuss and refer out for anti-inflammatory diet, sleeping modifications, reducing digital pollution, ice, heat and walking in nature.

Liz Durkin, OT

---

4. The vagus nerve is a major player in the body's handling of stress and there are theories about ways to impact the functioning of this nerve (the tone) for better stress coping.

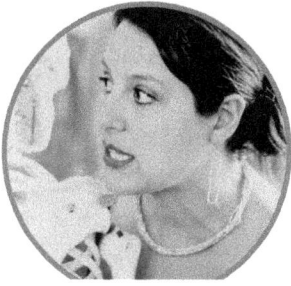

Richelle Ricard, LMT

I do. I believe in self-care, and I also know that nobody lives in a vacuum, so my treatments will not have long-lasting effects if they continue to live in their current state, constantly re-irritating the areas of focus. I often recommend Epsom salt baths/magnesium oil, extra sleep, owning and communicating their truths, dietary shifts, movement exercises, computer breaks, journaling. Baths and movement are the top two usually: dedicating time to Self is important, water element is powerful and magnesium is low for tons of folks. I also recommend movement and posture exercises as a simple way to start bringing more focused awareness to our body and thoughts; recognizing that we have habituated patterns in the physical realm can lead us to a productive questioning of "how and why" we do lots of things in our lives. Questioning leads to questing…

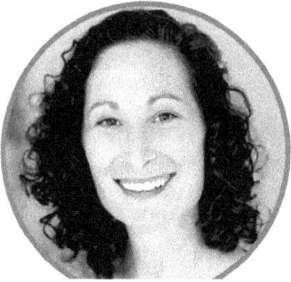

Heidi Gans, PT

Lately, my most common recommendation is for clients to take a moment, or a number of moments each day, to attune to bodily sensations, breath or posture. This allows them to check in and learn from the information offered by their physical bodies in each moment. The increased speed and quantity of mental stimulation in our modern world creates a sympathetic nervous system "bias," which agitates the body over time. Spending a few minutes focusing on some form of physiologic calming can make a significant difference in their experience. It does not take long.

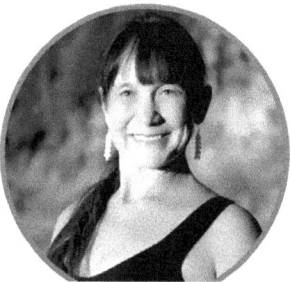

Michaelle Edwards

I recommend a diet of organic, unprocessed fresh foods with an emphasis on healthy organic greens and fats, no alcohol and lots of water. I would say that sitting less and walking more and eating an organic diet of fresh food is what I emphasize the most.

Ask the Pros

Are there any other common "homework" tasks (behavior modification) that you require of your patients/clients while under your care?

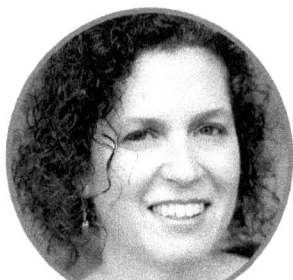

Not really.

Einat Arian, PhD, ND

Everyone I work with gets a home program. I usually ask for metrics on their engagement in these tasks, such as a journal to measure any changes such as duration or intensity.

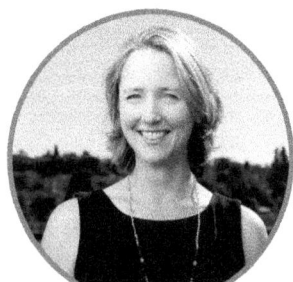

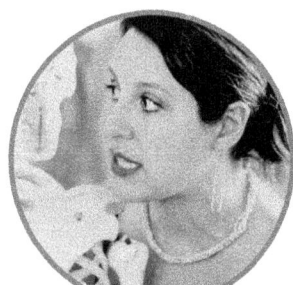

Susanne Michaud, DPT

Homework: mostly the above (lifestyle recommendations). But more specifically, I have been urging folks to look at how they align their feet when they stand or exercise. Most people have ingrained the idea that straight feet make for neutral alignment, but that just isn't the case. Individual bone differences often mean that for the hip to seat neutrally, the feet will point outward—sometimes quite a lot. Once that alignment has been achieved, the ankles, knees and low back are all in a much better alignment, set up for better stabilizing and muscular recruitment and at less risk for hypermobility/degeneration.

Richelle Ricard, LMT

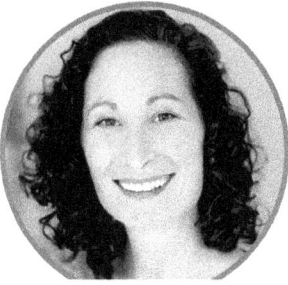

Heidi Gans, PT

Requiring clients to do things is not what I consider my role to be. Any task or exercise I recommend is posed as an "experiment," which a client can either choose to practice or not. For a week or two, I might ask a client to "trust me" and try something unfamiliar or new, but after that time, it must prove itself to be helpful. If a client tries an activity earnestly and diligently and gives it a good trial, then they will be able to evaluate for themselves whether it is worth continuing. The benefits should soon speak for themselves. If it works, it works.

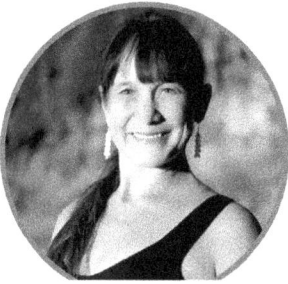

Michaelle Edwards

I recommend that clients sit in chairs with their hips 4 inches or more above the level of the knee and retain the natural curves of the spine in all static positions. They can use a yoga block or bolster, but they should always sit with the knees below the hips. I also recommend that people use an external keyboard if using a laptop computer to keep the head level with the rest of the spine. I ask people to practice safe forward bending by flexing the knees and moving the hips back when leaning over. I educate people on the anatomy of breathing and the benefits of pandiculation[5] over static stretching.

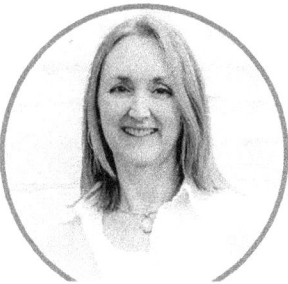

Liz Durkin, OT

Myofascial releases, breath work, walking, drinking water.

---

5. The term "pandiculation" when used in the context of somatics (body centered), is a way to describe a stretch that happens actively – meaning certain muscles are actively creating the elongation. This is in contrast with a simple "stretch" which is typically passive elongation.

Ask the Pros

Has there ever been a situation where you would turn someone away or redirect them to a different therapy/modality? If so, please explain the circumstances.

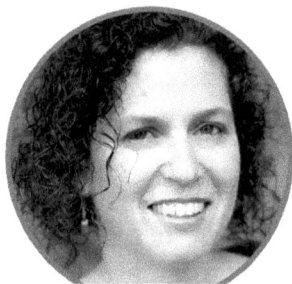

I want to see changes in the patient within 3 treatments; otherwise, the modality is probably not the right one.

I also want people to take responsibility for their own health and understand that it's unrealistic to expect me to "fix" them. They need to be active participants in finding solutions for their problems.

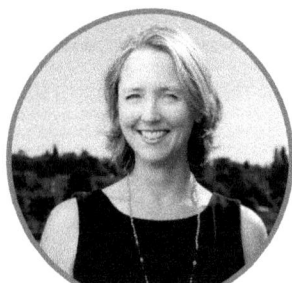

Einat Arian, PhD, ND

Absolutely. If my evaluation shows red flags that are not appropriate for PT, I direct them to their primary care providers. More often, though, I will have someone continue with a maintenance program after our bout of care is up, usually with massage, acupuncture or chiropractic. I believe physical therapy tune-ups should occur at least 2 times per year for general maintenance.

Susanne Michaud, DPT

However, these other passive modalities (massage, acupuncture or chiropractic) can occur more frequently given their endogenous opioid effects.[6,7]

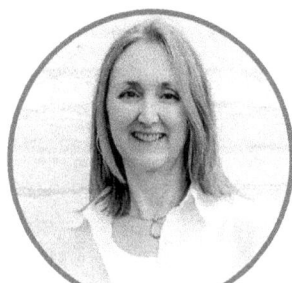

In my acupuncture practice, I have only turned away two clients, one whose injury was outside of my scope and another who was so uneasy about the energetic philosophy underlying acupuncture that I told her we did not have to continue. I have not turned away occupational therapy patients at an outpatient setting.

Liz Durkin, OT

---

6. "endogenous opioids" are molecules (neuropeptides) that the body can produce and release for pain relief.
7. Andrew D. Vigotsky, Ryan P. Bruhns, "The Role of Descending Modulation in Manual Therapy and Its Analgesic Implications: A Narrative Review", *Pain Research and Treatment*, vol. 2015, Article ID 292805, 11 pages, 2015. https://doi.org/10.1155/2015/292805

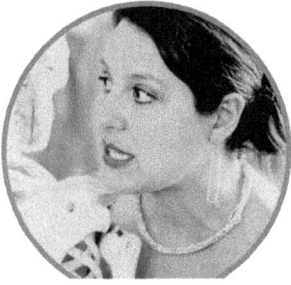

Richelle Ricard, LMT

I have turned folks toward other bodyworkers who specialize in modalities that I don't have the advanced skills in: neuro-fascial work, craniosacral. There have been a few cases of folks who were receiving multiple modalities, and due to their sensitive systems, this resulted in getting overtreated. In these cases, we discuss where they feel they are getting the most fruitful results and develop a plan to piggy-back one or the other at a later date, instead of working concurrently.

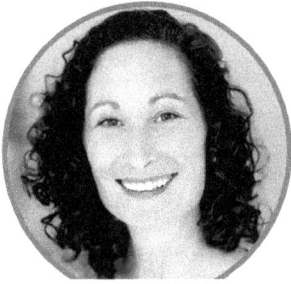

Heidi Gans, PT

If I believe my skills and tools are not appropriate or helpful for a client, I will freely send them on to others who might be more successful with them. I will also forward someone on if I feel they need care beyond the reach of my skill set.

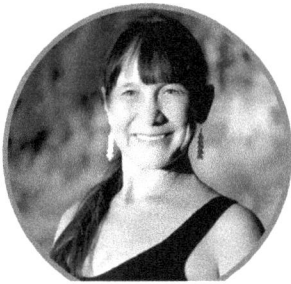

Michaelle Edwards

Chronic hip/back pain is something I have had a lot of success with. The techniques I teach my clients have an effect on all body systems at the nervous system level.

Ask the Pros

Is there a particular pain condition or variety of pain that you enjoy working with and/or have good success with? If so, please elaborate.

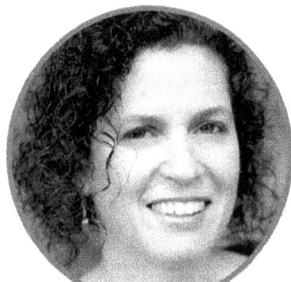

Einat Arian, PhD, ND

I like working with post-concussion patients, especially if some time has passed and they are still having symptoms.

People with disk syndromes can also really benefit from what I do.

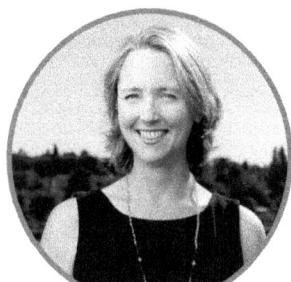

Susanne Michaud, DPT

Any musculoskeletal pain is welcome. I also work with many complicated cases where there is an autoimmune overlay to the pain, and that requires different pacing and approaches. I generally have great success with people who have radiculopathies[8] and peripheral nerve issues.

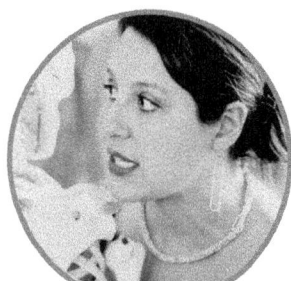

Richelle Ricard, LMT

I work with a ton of runners and athletes, who have a wide range of stuff to address. I think that lately the feet and legs are the focal point for addressing so many symptoms up stream. I'm also really intrigued by how the coccyx relates to both back and hip pain. The relationship between the feet and the tail bone is slowly becoming clearer to me; how we transfer gravity through the lower extremity and what are the most efficient ways to do so versus the most habitual ways.

---

8. "Radiculopathies" are pain conditions that follow a pain pattern often along the distribution of a nerve for example sciatica can manifest down the leg along the pathway of the sciatic nerve.

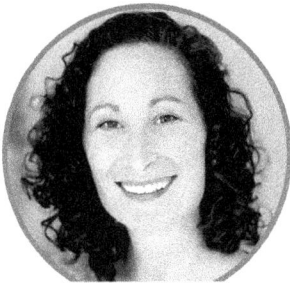

My stance has thus far been that "I treat whoever comes in the door."

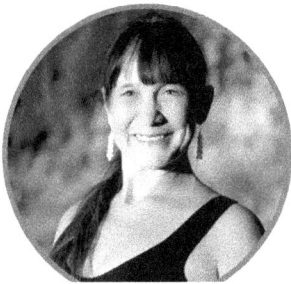

Heidi Gans, PT

Chronic hip/back pain is something I have had a lot of success with. The techniques I teach my clients have an effect on all body systems at the nervous system level.

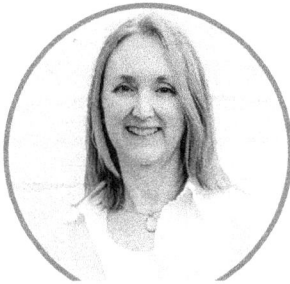

Michaelle Edwards

I am interested in working with chronic pain conditions related to Lyme's disease, Fibromyalgia, Epstein-Barr, Ehlers Danlos/hypermobility, and autoimmune disorders. Acupuncture and moxibustion[9] works extremely well for many autoimmune disorders and EBV/chronic fatigue. Recently, I have found that Bowen therapy has produced the best results of my career, perhaps because it is gentle, creating a parasympathetic response with simple moves and wait times that allow the nervous system to adjust to changes input through the fascial network/mechanoreceptors.[10]

Liz Durkin, OT

---

9. Moxibustion is a traditional Chinese medicine therapy which consists of burning dried mugwort on particular points on the body.
10. A sense organ or cell that responds to mechanical stimuli such as touch or sound.

Ask the Pros

Do you feel that your area of expertise (in regard to pain) relates in some way directly or indirectly to patients' experience of inflammation? If so, how?

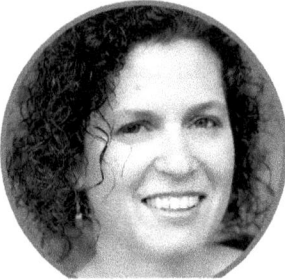

I think post-concussion syndromes have a lot to do with inflammation and even post-inflammation aftermath.

Disk syndromes are probably similar, but maybe less extreme.

I also think past inflammation can leave the nervous system "irritable" either locally or generally.

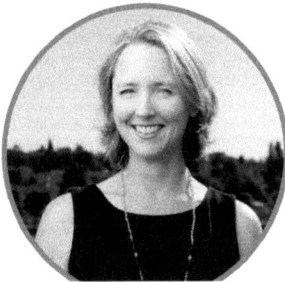

Einat Arian, PhD, ND

This is an interesting question. Inflammation is both a stew that many people live in based on their diets, environments or specific pathologies. But it is also a very important initial response to injury and trauma that is essential to the healing process. I find when someone in pain does not understand what is going on or has fear around what is happening, this can be the biggest hindrance to progress or improvement.

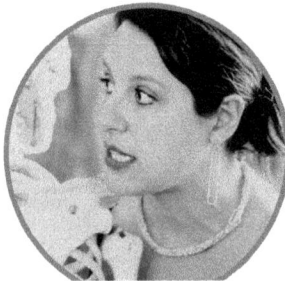

Susanne Michaud, DPT

Yes. The fascia-centered bodywork that I offer aims to create space between layers, to maximize the fluidity of the connective tissue, which provides better interstitial circulation and a more hospitable environment for the muscle, nerves, and organs to operate with less chemical stress around them. They can engage in a more efficient exchange of waste and fuel. Inflammation can do its rightful job without getting bogged down and becoming chronic or stagnant.

Richelle Ricard, LMT

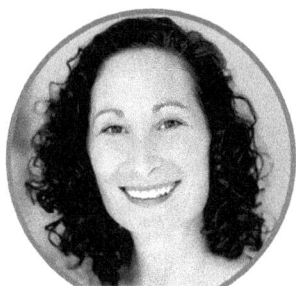

Heidi Gans, PT

I believe that pain, especially chronic pain, leads to a "hypervigilance" in the nervous system. My experience is that, if I successfully calm a person's nervous system, often globalized patterns of muscle guarding, bracing and pain will decrease. Inflammation in the body is meant to help by sending more resources to a given area; however, if a region or the nervous system itself is chronically in the inflamed state, it is hard to get clear feedback and information about the best way to move forward. Once the nervous system is calmed and superficial guarding patterns ease, it is much easier to have success with PT modalities, exercises and activities.

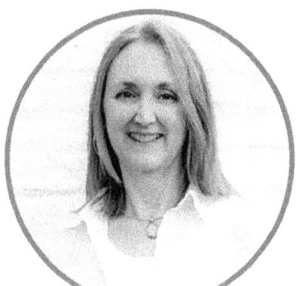

Liz Durkin, OT

My work is all about how to deal with inflammation, whether from poor diet, posture, infection, environmental pollution or lack of exercise. My way to decrease inflammation is multifactorial: through fascia, nervous system, diet, breath and movement.

Ask the Pros

Are there common misconceptions about your profession or your work that you encounter with patients? If so, how would you like to see/hear that clarified?

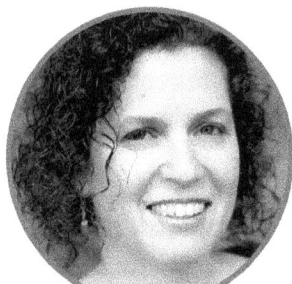

Sometimes people think Craniosacral therapy is mostly for the head. I feel that I work with the whole body through the fascia system both peripherally and in the head and spine as well as directly with the nervous system centrally but also along fascial restrictions around the nerves peripherally.

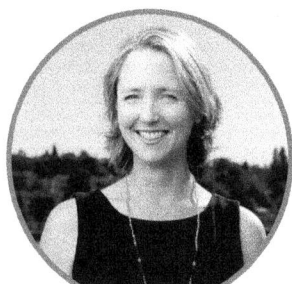

Einat Arian, PhD, ND

Many people think that all physical therapy is just exercise and that they can do this on their own. Exercise is a tool we use, but it is how we analyze the mechanics of a person's movement that targets how an exercise can be either healthful or harmful. Assessing and prescribing movements that target a person's individual issues is how we use exercise. In addition, we give people many self-corrective tools to mitigate alignment and movement dysfunction. When these do not work, we use manual therapy and neuromuscular techniques to affect change.

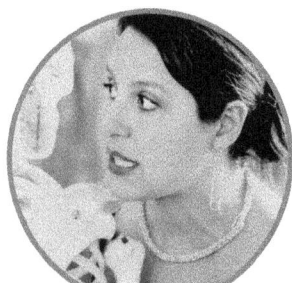

Susanne Michaud, DPT

Oh yes, but they are too varied to mention. Overall, massage is still seen by most as a spa treatment. The relaxation response is certainly a valid reason to receive this work, but it's still a minority of the population who views massage as a legitimate treatment for long-term relief from acute or chronic conditions. We need to do a better job at sharing with the masses that there are vast and varied approaches to bodywork that really can address the whole person, while also focusing on specific ailments.

Richelle Ricard, LMT

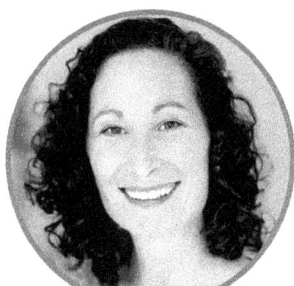

I think many physical therapists rely on routines, repetition and protocols, which is partly due to the restrictions of third-party payers. However, I will often hear a client say, "my last PT did not really hear me. They just gave me a set of exercises, which did not really help much." Many clients call me a "non-traditional" PT, which is less about the techniques and tools I use and

Heidi Gans, PT

more about my willingness to address what motivates and inspires them to heal. As PTs, I feel we have a unique opportunity to form important relationships and connections with our clients so that we can move together towards less pain, higher function and improved life experience.

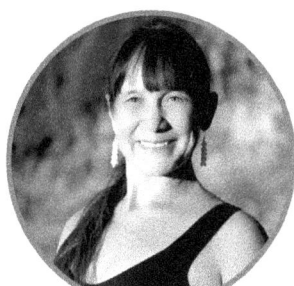

The word "yoga" makes most people think that I teach some kind of static stretching or poses as in traditional yoga. YogAlign, the style of yoga and self-guided bodywork that I created, is not :stretching" but is more about the global balancing of tensional forces in the body. Anyone can do it as it is based on posture rather than yoga pose alignment.

Michaelle Edwards

I have been actively educating people to avoid the liabilities of too much flexibility. The yoga industry has glamorized hyper-flexibility and led people to focus too much on performance of yoga poses rather than posture alignment for daily living.

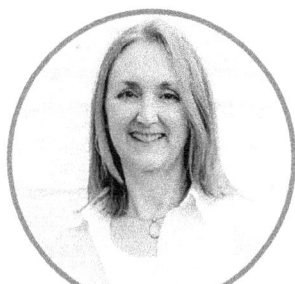

Acupuncture: that it hurts (doesn't have to), that it is magical (it is, but there is a lot of scientific evidence for its mechanisms) and that it takes only a few treatments (it works best when used preventatively/seasonally). Occupational Therapy: that we only treat the upper extremities. In our clinic, we treat the whole body and provide unique global and systems perspectives.

Liz Durkin, OT

The Take-Aways

➤ An important piece to the experience of any modality is to be shown a way to experience a glimmer of hope …a moment of being pain-free to remind yourself that it's possible.

➤ Find practitioners who will be a sounding board for you and who can help clarify your needs and the path forward for your individual situation.

➤ There seems to be consensus that it takes a village and not any single modality can be the magic bullet. But there also needs to be moderation with frequency and volume of intervention. One thing at a time and with room in between to let the body rest and process changes.

➤ Sleep, stress management or mitigation, breathing and eating, are things that we all agree will support treatment progress.

➤ Many of us providers take oaths to open our doors to anyone and everyone but it's natural to develop special interests and strengths for certain types of clinical cases. It's a completely fair question as a patient to inquire about this when interviewing a prospective healthcare provider.

➤ Impacting inflammation can happen through many different avenues but there seems to be some consensus that doing so is directly and indirectly part of care when pain is at play.

➤ As a patient, it might be useful to set aside preconceived notions about certain disciplines of healthcare because no two practitioners deliver the same experience of human interaction. The therapeutic relationship can be as unique as each human being.

Hopefully these interviews offer you a snapshot of the vast array of modalities that can address your body mechanics. But also, that the reach is wider than just body mechanics.

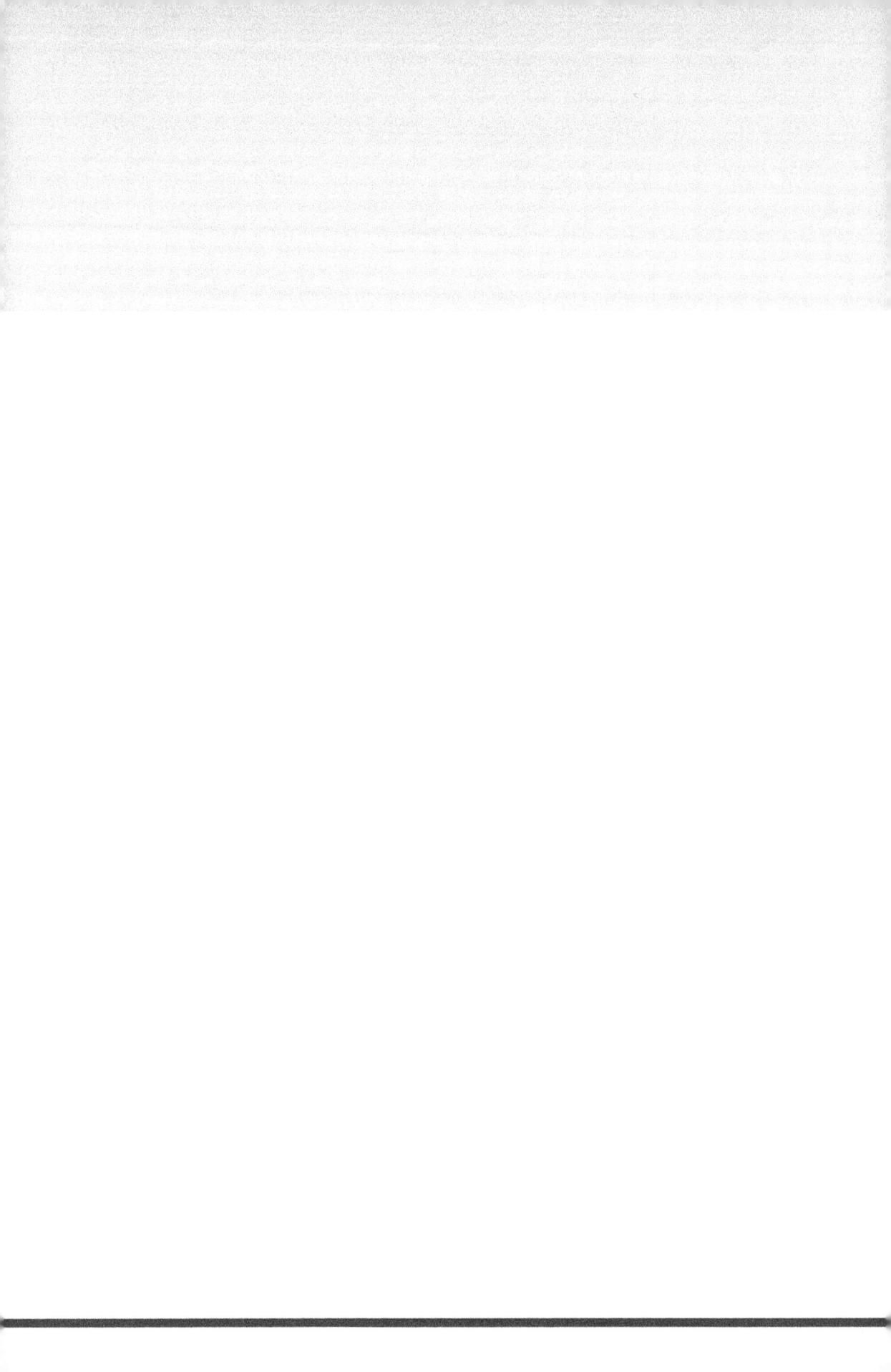

MAKE THE MOST OF YOUR VISIT

Questions to ask when checking out new practitioners to aid with biomechanical reinforcement:

1. How do you see your role in this process?

2. What are your expectations of me?

3. Is there a timeline with milestones to reach for?

4. How do you measure progress and when do I know it's time to move on?

5. How often do you see and work with clinical cases like mine?

A few things you should prepare to share with your practitioners:

1. Communicate your pain with as many descriptive adjectives as possible.

2. Pay attention to the situations and time of day when you notice your pain the most.

3. Remember and share with your provider which of the Action Plan activities provided relief.

ABOUT THE AUTHOR

YA-LING J. LIOU, DC, is a chiropractic physician who, after more than 30 years of clinical experience, continues to expand and share her intuitive body care techniques. All of her work takes into account the whole person, aiming not only to address the mechanical balance of the body, but also the chemical and emotional aspects that so often influence this balance.

Growing up with exposure to generations of Eastern as well as Western attitudes toward health has provided Dr. Liou with a unique perspective on health care. She began her formal education in the area of applied sciences in her hometown of Montreal, Quebec, before completing a degree program at New York Chiropractic College.

Dr. Liou now lives, works, and writes in Seattle. She taught anatomy, physiology and kinesiology at Seattle Massage School (currently Everest College and formerly Ashmead College) and later brought her multiple-systems perspective to the Naturopathic Physical Medicine Department at Bastyr University as an adjunct faculty member.

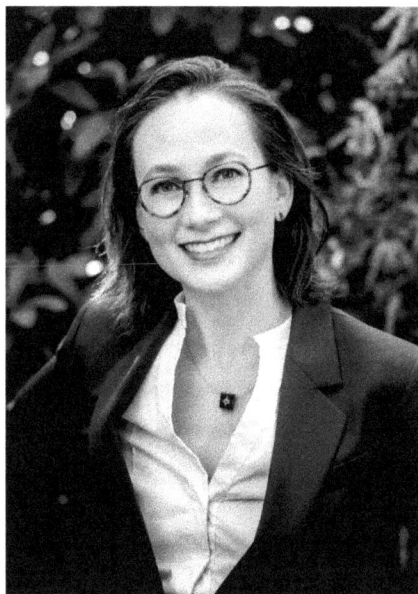

Want to learn more? Stay connected with the author by visitng www.ya-ling.com.

www.ingramcontent.com/pod-product-compliance
Lightning Source LLC
Chambersburg PA
CBHW051323020426

42333CB00032B/3459